WHISPERS FROM ETERNITY

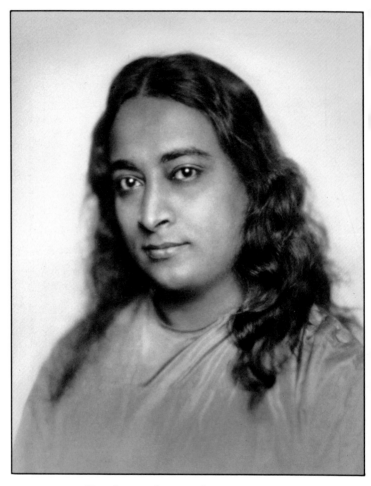

"Read my *Whispers from Eternity* —
eternally through it I will talk to you."

—Paramahansa Yogananda

Whispers from Eternity

BY

PARAMAHANSA YOGANANDA

Foreword by Amelita Galli-Curci

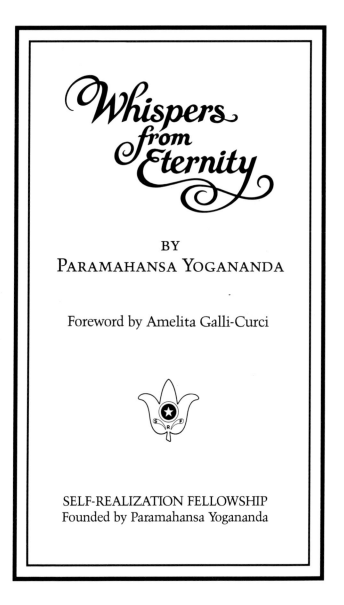

SELF-REALIZATION FELLOWSHIP
Founded by Paramahansa Yogananda

Authorized by the International Publications Council of Self-Realization Fellowship

Self-Realization Fellowship was founded in 1920 by Paramahansa Yogananda as the instrument for the worldwide dissemination of his teachings. The reader may be certain of the authenticity of publications by or about Paramahansa Yogananda and his teachings if the registered Self-Realization emblem, and/or the statement of authorization (shown together above), appears on those works.

Printed in the United States of America

ISBN 0–87612–100–8
ISBN 0–87612–103–2 (illustrated)
Library of Congress Catalog Number: 86–060584
10611–5

Dedicated unto
Christians, Moslems, Buddhists, Hebrews,
Hindus, and all other religionists,
In whom the Cosmic Heart is ever throbbing
equally

And unto
The multicolored lamps of various true
teachings,
In which shines the same white flame of God

And unto
All churches, mosques, viharas, tabernacles,
pagodas, and temples of the world,
Wherein the One Father dwells impartially
in the fullness of His glory

CONTENTS

Acknowledgments viii
Publisher's Note ix
Foreword, by Amelita Galli-Curci xi
Introduction xiii

SECTION I
Prayers and Soul Thoughts 1

SECTION II
Invocations to the Manifestations of God in
    the Temples of Great Lives 125

SECTION III
Children's Prayers 139

SECTION IV
Experiences in Superconsciousness 149

Paramahansa Yogananda: A Yogi in Life
    and Death 200
Aims and Ideals of Self-Realization Fellowship ... 202
Glossary 203
Alphabetical Index of Titles 217

*   *   *

Photographs of Paramahansa Yogananda

The author (frontispiece)
At Niagara Falls, New York, 1927 41
At Encinitas, California, 1938 88
In 1926 150

ACKNOWLEDGMENTS

The paintings used in *Whispers from Eternity* have been reproduced with the kind permission and co-operation of several museums, galleries, and individuals:

Page 12: Detail from "The Girl and the Dog," by Theodore Robinson. Cincinnati Art Museum, Cincinnati, Ohio. Gift of Mrs. A. M. Adler.

Page 28: Detail from "An Angel Adoring," by Filippino Lippi. Reproduced by courtesy of the Trustees, The National Gallery, London.

Pages 36–37: Detail from "The Voyage of Life: Old Age," by Thomas Cole. National Gallery of Art, Washington, D.C.; Ailsa Mellon Bruce Fund.

Page 55: "Do Unto Others," by Norman Rockwell. © 1961 Estate of Norman Rockwell. Used by permission.

Page 68: "Christ at the Sea of Galilee," by Jacopo Tintoretto. National Gallery of Art, Washington, D.C.; Samuel H. Kress Collection.

Page 94: "The Voyage of Life: Manhood," by Thomas Cole. National Gallery of Art, Washington, D.C.; Ailsa Mellon Bruce Fund.

Page 142: "A Girl with a Watering Can," by Auguste Renoir. National Gallery of Art, Washington, D.C.; Chester Dale Collection.

Page 191: Detail (angel) from "The Virgin of the Rocks," by Leonardo da Vinci. Reproduced by courtesy of the Trustees, The National Gallery, London.

PUBLISHER'S NOTE

Since Paramahansa Yogananda's *Autobiography of a Yogi* was first published in 1946, his writings have received recognition in all parts of the world—from the literary and general public as well as from his followers. It is therefore not surprising that there are now a number of other publishers, organizations, and individuals claiming to represent his teachings. Some are borrowing the name of this beloved world teacher to further their own societies or interests, or to gain recognition for themselves. Others are presenting what are purported to be his "original" teachings, but what is in fact material taken from publications that had been poorly edited by temporary helpers or compiled from incomplete notes taken during Paramahansa Yogananda's classes. The Guru was very dissatisfied with the presentation of this material, and later did much work on it and gave specific instructions for its correction and clarification.

During the closing years of his life, Paramahansaji also revised *Whispers from Eternity.* In an "Author's Note" written in 1951 for inclusion in his revised edition of this book, he said:

> It has given me great satisfaction to revise *Whispers from Eternity.* When first published, the book contained unedited writings and a number of verbatim transcripts of prayers composed by me in my yoga classes in various cities.

> For many years I wished to edit these invocations but was prevented by the pressure of other duties. During the last three years I have taken time now and then to revise the book.
>
> I am immensely grateful to a Self-Realization Fellowship student who gave me invaluable aid in the work of editing, revision, and rearrangement.*

Readers sometimes inquire how they can be sure that a publication accurately presents the life and teachings of Sri Yogananda. In response to these inquiries, we would like to explain that Paramahansa Yogananda founded Self-Realization Fellowship in 1920 to be the instrument for worldwide dissemination of his teachings. He personally chose and trained those close disciples who constitute the Self-Realization Fellowship Publications Council, giving them specific guidelines for the publishing of his writings, lectures, and *Self-Realization Lessons.* The presence in a publication of the emblem shown on page *ix,* or the statement, "Authorized by the International Publications Council of Self-Realization Fellowship," assures the reader of the authenticity of that work.

* Sentiment for the first version of Paramahansaji's *Whispers from Eternity* has persisted among some of his devoted followers. A "First Version" edition is published by and available from Self-Realization Fellowship.

FOREWORD

The prayers in *Whispers from Eternity* serve to bring God closer to us, by describing the liberating feelings that arise from actual communion with Him.

The Lord is here portrayed in His immanent aspect: the Cosmic Mother—a grand conception of the Infinite and Invisible become, in Nature, finite and visible.

Followers of all religions may drink from this fountain of universal prayers. Paramahansa Yogananda's writings give profound answers to questions of the modern scientific mind, seeking God intelligently.

The book offers a great variety of invocations, enabling the truth seeker to choose daily the thought most helpful to his particular need.

I make this humble request to the reader:

"Pass not by, with hurried intellectual reading, the precious mines of truth hidden in the soil of words in this sacred book. Instead, dig deep in the mines with the pickax of attentive, reverent, and meditative study; and finally find the priceless gem of Self-realization."

AMELITA GALLI-CURCI

INTRODUCTION

I offer my simple songs at the shrine of humanity, that all share my soul joy. May the Spirit in these devotional outpourings restore in many men the wilting blossom of high aspiration.

In naming the book *Whispers from Eternity* I mean, by Eternity, God in the aspect of the Eternal Mother. In the Lord's transcendent aspect, the Absolute, He is unreachable by human thought; but in His immanent aspect—permeating the atoms of the universal structure, externalizing Himself in man and Nature—He is near and approachable, the Refuge and Redeemer of every creature.

In the Hindu scriptures His immanence is symbolized as the Mother that presides with watchful love over the destinies of countless beings and over the developments of the endless cycles of creation.*

It is this personalized aspect of the Ultimate Reality that may be said to have "longings" for the rightful behavior of Her children and to answer gladly their prayers.

Those who imagine that the Impersonal cannot manifest Itself in a personal form are in effect denying Its omnipotence and the possibility that man can commune with his Maker. The Lord has often appeared in living tangibility before true *bhaktas* (devo-

---

* See pages 178-181 and *yugas* in glossary.

tees of a personal God). Down the ages He has materialized Himself before the gaze of His devotees in whatever forms they hold most dear. A Christian sees Jesus, a Moslem sees Mohammed, a Hindu sees Krishna or Rama,* and so on.

The Lord yearns to behold each man playing perfectly his given role on earth. It is by misuse of free will that human beings thwart the divine plan. Absence of the clamor of egotistical desires enables us to hear and heed the guiding Voice within. Free from self-will, men of wisdom carry on their activities in effortless accordance with God's design.

"Not as I will, but as Thou wilt," Jesus prayed. No karma* accrues to the man who rightfully enacts his part in the drama of earthly life.

Divine recollection is the simplest way to achieve God-communion. Our inner assertion of spiritual identity is sufficient to operate the law for fulfillment of prayers. This law has been utilized by saints of all lands. From the depths of his own experience, Christ was able to give us this glorious assurance:

"If ye have faith, and doubt not…if ye shall say unto this mountain, Be thou removed, and be thou cast into the sea, it shall be done. And all things whatsoever ye shall ask in prayer, believing, ye shall receive."†

Supplications to the Indwelling Spirit should be made with intense fervor. They will be answered by soul whispers — silent mysterious responses that quickly transform one's life.

Devotees who, with closed eyes, repeat over and over the affirmations in this book, trying to feel their

* See glossary.
† Matthew 21:21-22.

deep truths, will *spiritualize* them; that is, rouse their inspiration slumbering beneath the thick silken quilt of words.

Invocations to the Lord are like ever-living plants that ceaselessly put forth new blossoms. The prayer plants in *Whispers from Eternity* retain the same branches of words; yet, if watered by the divine dew of meditation, each plant will daily yield fresh soul flowers of inexhaustibly varied insights.

SECTION I

―――――

PRAYERS AND
SOUL THOUGHTS

Salutation to God as the Great Preceptor
(Sanskrit scriptures)

Full of bliss, bestowing joy transcendent, Essence of wisdom, untouched by duality,* clear as the taintless sky, the utterer of *Thou art That*, the One, eternal, pure, immovable, the omnipresent Witness, free from Nature's three qualities,† beyond the reach of thought—my Divine Preceptor, I bow to Thee!

The melody of human brotherhood

Heavenly Spirit, we are traveling by many right roads to Thine abode of light. Guide us onto the highway of Self-knowledge, to which all paths of true religious beliefs eventually lead.

The diverse religions are branches of Thy one immeasurable tree of truth. May we enjoy the luscious fruits of soul realization that hang from the boughs of scriptures of every clime and time.

Teach us to chant in harmony the countless expressions of our supreme devotion. In Thy temple of the earth, in a chorus of many-accented voices, we are singing only to Thee.

O Divine Mother, lift us on Thy lap of universal love. Break Thy vow of silence and sing to us the heart-melting melody of human brotherhood.

* See *maya* in glossary.   † See *gunas* in glossary.

4

We unite to worship Thee, O Spirit! To worship Thee, O Spirit, with a myriad living thoughts of devotion we have built a universal shrine—domeless, immeasurable. In reverence niches we place lustrous wisdom lamps from all temples, tabernacles, viharas,* pagodas,* mosques, and churches.

The commingled incense of our divine yearnings soars in spirals from the bowl of our hearts. In the unutterable language of love we pour out to Thee our paeans of praise.

Within our silenced beings the mighty organ of *Aum* plays the canticle of all aspirations, the lament of all tears, and the swelling shout of all joys.

In this wall-less soul structure we, Thy children, are united. We feel the grace of Thy pleasure, O Father of All! *Amen, Hum, Amin, Aum.* *

* See glossary.

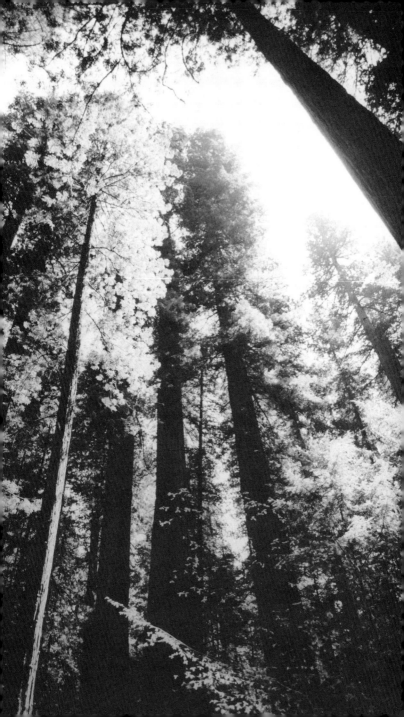

May I O Lord of Compassion, teach
forgive all me to shed tears of love for all
beings. May I behold them as
my very own—different expressions of my Self.

I easily excuse my own faults; let me therefore quickly forgive the failings of others. Bless me, O Father, that I not inflict on my companions unwelcome criticism. If they ask my advice in trying to correct themselves, may I offer suggestions inspired by Thee.

Through the strength of kindness and love, free from the thought of compulsion, teach me to lead all stumbling and stubborn ones to Thee. Guide my understanding and powers, that I turn dark-natured beings into sparkling seers who fully reflect Thy wisdom rays.

As even to a hanged murderer Thou dost give a fresh opportunity for self-improvement in a new incarnation, in which he wears an unrecognizable body and moves in another environment, so may my pity extend to world-forsaken wrongdoers. O Spirit, let the warmth of my love melt the chill in error-frozen brothers!

Thou art meekly waiting to reveal to all men Thy presence within them. O Unparalleled Patience, silent before an indifferent world! bestow on me Thy greathearted forbearance. Let me never retaliate when people wound me with unkindness.

May I sympathetically help others to help themselves. Teach me not to condemn their ingratitude if they turn against me and no longer permit me to serve them.

May I forgive (first inwardly, then outwardly) those who have most deeply injured me. I would return love for hatred, sweet praise for sour complaints, and good for evil.

Thy divine light is hidden in even the most vicious and gloom-shrouded man, waiting to shine forth under the proper conditions: the keeping of good company, and ardent desires for self-betterment.

We thank Thee that no sin is unforgivable, no evil insuperable; for the world of relativity does not contain absolutes.

Direct me, O Heavenly Father, that I awaken Thy bewildered ones to the consciousness of their native purity, immortality, and celestial sonhood.

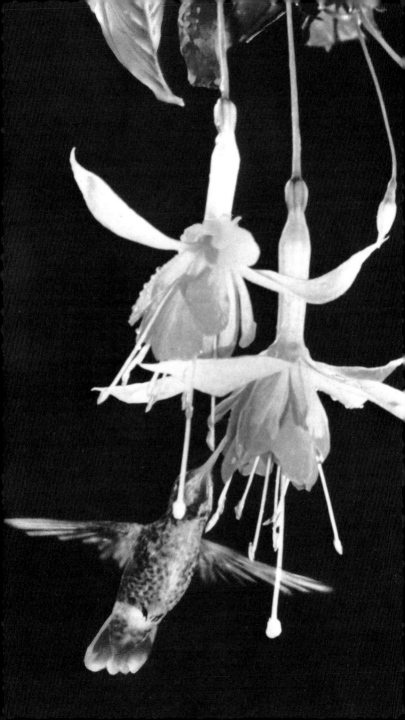

I am Thy tiny hummingbird

I am Thy tiny hummingbird, whirring with Thy power and ever searching for Thee.

I am Thy tiny humming-bird, darting afar to discover Thy rarest blooms; and to revel on high mountain crags in Thy color symphonies.

I am Thy tiny hummingbird, creating by my swiftness the hum that is praise of Thy Name.

I am Thy tiny hummingbird, dipping my beak into the hearts of life's multicolored flowers. May Thy grace prevent my tasting any poison plants of evil.

I am Thy tiny hummingbird, sipping nectar from blossoms in humble wayside plots of human sweetness and in Thy secret gardens of glory.

Give me the humblest place within Thy heart

O Creator of All! in the garden of Thy dreams let me be a radiant flower. Or may I be a tiny star, held on the timeless thread of Thy love as a twinkling bead in the vast necklace of Thy heavens.

Or give me the highest honor: the humblest

place within Thy heart. There I would behold the creation of the noblest visions of life.

O Master Weaver of Dreams, teach me to loom a cushioning carpet of Self-realization on which all Thy lovers may tread as they travel to the shrine of eternal wakefulness.

May I join the worshiping angels who offer at Thine altar the bouquets of their ever new perceptions and intuitions of Thee.

May I act from free choice, not habit

Teach me, O Father, to seek the soul's lasting happiness rather than temporary sense pleasures.

Strengthen my will power, that I escape from bad habits and reform myself by meditation and the influence of spiritually minded companions.

Give me the wisdom to follow happily the ways of righteousness. May I develop the soul faculty of discrimination that detects evil, in even its subtlest forms; and that guides me to the humble paths of goodness.

I would direct my life by the God-given power of free choice, not by the compulsions of hardened habits.

I yearn to hear Thy unique voice

Manifest Thyself to me, O Spirit, as the Source of all wisdom. Reveal to me the mystery of Thine incessant dance in protons and electrons.

Speak to me in the sound of *Aum,* * Thy cosmic vibration that commanded creation to spring forth, that empowered each atom to sing a distinctive note.

O August Primeval, deeply I yearn to hear Thy unique voice!

May I love Thee as saints love Thee

O Heavenly Father, fill me daily with the love and thanksgiving that overwhelm the heart of a newly awakened saint. Give me the fervor known to all devotees who have ever loved and found Thee.

* See glossary.

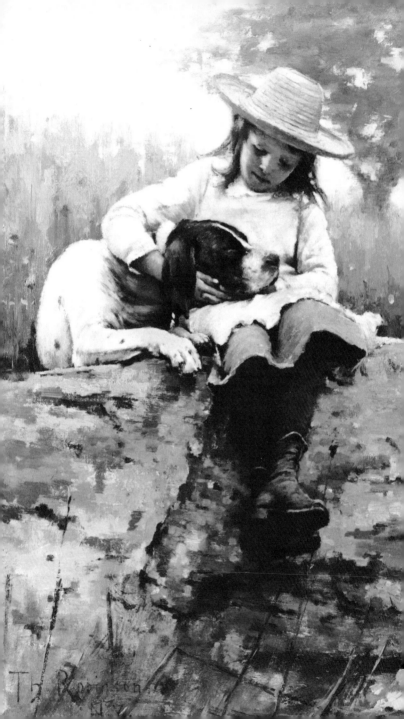

May human love become divine love

O Cosmic Mother, teach me to use the gift of Thy love in my heart to expand endlessly my sympathies.

May I pass from the boundaries of family affections into a larger realm of friendship and service to all. Let me not tarry, fascinated by rewarding feelings of usefulness, in even those noble regions—the farthest reaches of human solicitude.

Inspire me to enter the infinitudes of divine love. O Universal Spirit, I would invisibly embrace as my own all animate and seemingly inanimate forms in creation.

May I perceive even in stones, built of Thy secret atoms, the pulsing of Thine insuppressible life.

An ever present Sentry of Light

Let me give the divine opiate of Thy peace to groaning hearts, that they find sweet rest in Thee.

May I be a sudden sun-smile to all dreary natures; a fertility rain to arid minds; and a gift of kindness to the ill-treated: an ever present Sentry of Light, chasing away the thief, Gloom.

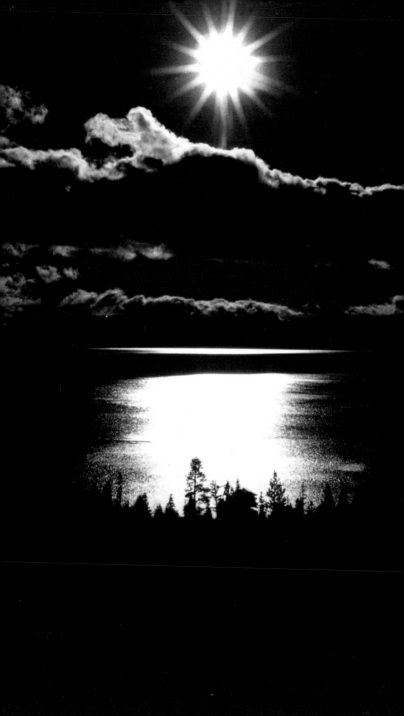

Thy light transfigures all creation

O Transubstantial Light! Thou art unseen, imperceptible, whether in warm rays of the sun or in cool moonbeams. The skyey lamps disclose only Dame Nature, not Thee.

The world of matter revealed by gross luminaries is but darkness to me. Train my vision to see Thy hidden effulgence, transfiguring the whole of creation.

When I sit with eyes closed, enveloped in self-created shadows, cause Thou to blaze upon me in splendor the aurora of intuition.* With worshiping gaze may I watch Thee in Thy ritual dance of cosmic activities.

The star that leads to the Christ Child

O Lord, I have long been engrossed in material things. Enthralled by their outward forms, I failed to perceive within them Thy creative Spirit. The starry single eye† of my soul insight is now being opened. Through it may I behold creation ashine with Thy glory.

Bless me, that I ever see the Eastern† star of wisdom. May it gleam before my human eyes, alike in daylight and in gloom.

Let my wise thoughts follow the wondrous star that leads to the Christ Child of Infinity.

* See glossary.   † See *spiritual eye* in glossary.

Give me fervor in divine love

O Spirit, teach me to worship Thee as wholeheartedly as a miser idolizes money. Let me be as deeply attached to Thee as a drunkard is to wine. May I cling to Thee as stubbornly as erring ones adhere to their bad habits. Inspire me to crave Thee as a worldly man yearns for possessions.

I long to be as attentive to Thee as a mother to her newborn babe. Lead me to seek Thee with the self-abandonment of Thy greatest devotees.

O Adored of the Angels, with the first fervor of true lovers may I cherish Thee ever!

Prayer before meditation

O Father, I cleanse the shrine of my heart with the holy waters of repentance. My bold passions, my long-sheltered ignorance, tremblingly await sacrifice upon Thine altar.

My little prayers arouse themselves in reverence, expecting Thee. My little joys dance in harmony with the temple bells of the far-flung spheres.

The muffled drum of my craving beats deep for Thee. I repeat Thy Name on mystic beads, fashioned of my crystal teardrops and polished with my love for Thee. Come, Spirit, come!

Save me from sense slavery   O Pristine Spirit of Purity! save me from insatiable sense cravings. Let my greedy desires be reduced to dross in a white heat of wisdom. By stern non-cooperation may I control all unruliness of the senses. Guide me to cooperate only with Thy will, harmoniously playing my little note, performing my little deed, singing my little song.

Inspire me to use the senses only in wholesome ways; and to discipline them wisely, that they desire to contribute to my true happiness. Lead them to conform joyously to Thy plan for them: freshness, acuity, irreproachableness.

As electricity may either illuminate or destroy a building, so man's powers may glorify or devastate his life. Teach me, then, to employ rightly the sensory energies Thou hast entrusted to me.

Transmute my sense craving into soul craving. And, O Spirit! let me feel Thy rod of discipline if ever I stray senseward away from Thee.

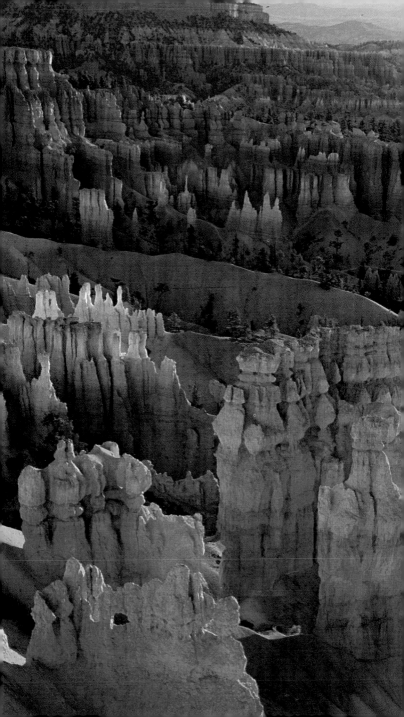

**O Spirit,
I worship
Thee in
all shrines**
Into the temple of peace come Thou, O Lord of Joy! Enter my shrine of meditation, O Bliss God! Sanctify me with Thy presence.

Eternal Allah,* hover over the lone minaret of my holy aspiration. The mosque of my mind exudes a frankincense of stillness.

On the altar of my inner vihara* I place flowers of desirelessness. Their chaste beauty is Thine, O Spirit!

In a tabernacle not made with hands, I bow before the sacred ark and vow to keep Thy commandments.

Heavenly Father, in an invisible church built of devotion granite, receive Thou my humble heart offerings, daily renewed by prayer.

**In appearance,
many; in
essence, One**
O Eternal Fire, Thou art shooting a little soul flame of individual human consciousness through each pore in the Great Burner of Thy Universal Mind. Thou dost appear many, limited, small, divided, in these separate soul fires; but all are projections of Thy One Infinite Flame.

* See glossary.

Inspirit us with generosity

Heavenly Father, inspirit us with generosity. Thy Being is an outpouring of bounty; let us, too, know the joy of giving.

Teach us to spend for others' necessities as naturally as for our own. Since we shudder at even the thought of destitution for ourselves, may we sympathetically help those who in actuality know the pangs of want.

Let us realize that to die rich, without having shared our treasures, is to die poor in Thine eyes; and to die poor because of liberality is to die rich with Thy blessings.

Men selfishly blinded by opulence must experience poverty in this or a future earth-life, because in the abodes of the world-abandoned they saw Thee not.

In all experiences of Thy children it is Thine omnipresent consciousness that enjoys and suffers. Thou didst bestow riches on Thyself (in the forms of the wealthy) as an intricate human test to see how charitable Thou wouldst be to Thyself (in the forms of the needy).

The largehearted man, receiving from Thee loving largess and freely bestowing it on others, expands into the Universal Self.

Accepting daily Thine endless gifts, may we praise Thee and thank Thee, O Giver of All!

Tell me—
wilt Thou
be mine?

I care not if I have to endure all pains, and relinquish every earthly desire—if in the end I find Thee!

I mind not if I must pass through sextillions of lives, undergoing the throes of birth and the pangs of death; leaving behind me a heap of my mangled fleshly forms—if at last I find Thee!

Lord, tell me Thou wilt surely be mine! Then, realizing the immensity of Thy gift of Thyself and the littleness of any gift or sacrifice I could make in return, I shall patiently pass through a hundred thousand years as though they were but a day.

Tell me—*wilt Thou be mine!*

The untutored
song of
my heart

I sing a hymn unuttered by any other voice. To Thee I offer the virgin theme that my heart chants secretly. Alone I have nurtured my song child; now I bring it to Thee for Thy training.

To Thee I give no intellectual, premeditated, and disciplined aria; only the untutored strains of my heart. For Thee no hothouse flowers, watered by careful emotions; only rare wild blossoms that grow spontaneously on the highest tracts of my soul.

Thou art ever busy, O Cosmic Potter! Heavenly Father, we thank Thee for sharing with all creatures and natural forces Thy responsibilities in carrying on the work of creation. May we, Thy human children, never complain of our tasks.

Dost Thou not keep the bee busy? and the animals, providing for their young? and the dark water-wagons of the sky, sprinkling rain on thirsty greens?

The amoeba, the whippoorwill, and gigantic fiery-eyed planets, growling in the forest of space—all are performing some of Thy work.

O Alert Lord, busiest of all! noting the fall of a sparrow, attending the slightest scratch of flesh, and coursing the path of meteors.

With vibratory fingers didst Thou mold earth's clay ball; daily Thou art whirling it, ray-strung to the sun and rhythmically revolving around it.

O Cosmic Potter, on Thy wheel of life Thou dost form trillions of never-duplicated vessels of flesh — vulnerable vehicles of man's immortal Spirit.

Thine unseen creation factory produces *every-thing* — all furnishings and equipment needed by Thy sons for their physical, mental, and spiritual mansions.

Thou art the Originator, Manufacturer, and ever timely Exhibitor of "Nature Products." Thou art the Celestial Salesman who extols the value of new inner possessions for the fine art of gracious living.

Thy cooperative plan requires that for Thy bounties man offer payment. He must give money or labor in the soil to obtain nourishing food; he must observe carefulness and moderation to maintain health; he must proffer coins of study and self-improvement to receive sufficient currents of light and power for his cozy mental cottage. And he must dig diligently within to discover the spring of devotional waters that will purify him for Thy coming.

All material things may be bought and sold; but Thou, O Priceless One, art not for sale!

Each of Thy children will someday "come to Himself," realizing his divine status. Then inexhaustible bliss descends as Thy grace, forever freely given.

**A river
of ardor**
To meet Thee I am rushing forward on a river of ardor made of crystal tears of my cravings for Thee. Wilt Thou channel the boisterous waters, that they be not lost in a desert of disappointment? Wilt Thou see that my mad flood of devotion follows the right course, straight to Thee?

**Make me clean
again, Divine
Mother**
Thou didst dress me in raiment immaculate, and sent me out to play. I wandered away and frolicked among the fruitless trees of delusion. The shadows of the forest of suffering enveloped me.

I went out spotless; now I am besmirched with the mud of ignorance. O Divine Mother, wash me in waters of Thy wisdom! Make me clean again!

**Crying in the
wilderness**
I am crying in the wilderness of my loneliness. Eyes closed in prayer, long have I scanned inner skies of darkness to discover the hidden light of Thy presence.

With countless heart cravings I pant for Thy raindrops of wisdom. Relieve my thirst, O Ever Flowing Waters!

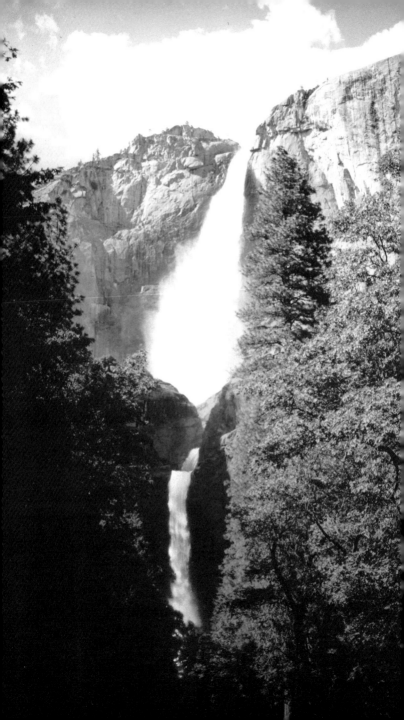

Thou art visible as Mother Nature Unborn and Beginningless, Unfathomable Infinite! remote, inapprehensible by mortals, Thou art near and dear to them in Thine aspect of Form and Finitude—Mother Nature. Through Her starry eyes man may gaze into the threshold of Thine innocent Mystery.

O Lady of Loveliness! Thy vast skyey garments are ever, never the same: tender glow of dawn, dazzling rays of midday, transitional tones of dusk, and enigma veil of darkness.

I gaze raptly on Thy face, blazing by day with the sun's vital power and bestowing by night soothing moonbeam glances. I mix my breath with Thine in the heaving winds. I feel Thy cosmic energy in the pulse of my being, and hear Thy footsteps in the tread of all creatures.

I watch Thy hands at work in the law of gravitation; and reflect, awestruck, on Thine activities in electromagnetic waves. I behold the pores of the skies perspiring with Thy strenuous life, showering the potent rains; and see Thy bloodstream flowing red in the veins of men, crystal clear in brooklets, and transparent blue in oceans.

O Voice of Silent Spirit, O Divine Ventriloquist! Thine echoes come to me in the sound of blown conchs, the drumbeat of marching seas, the gossip of birds, and the secret hum* of vibrations.

Orientwise, with dueful ceremony I worship Thee, O Goddess of Endless Giving! In the temple of my mind I ring bells of harmony, place on the altar flowers of devotion, and set alight blessed thought candles and the incense of love.

O my Cosmic Idol, diademed with the rainbow, garlanded with stringèd pearls of the Milky Way, and wearing on Thy fingers diamonds of glittering planets, to Thee I bow!

* See *Aum* in glossary.

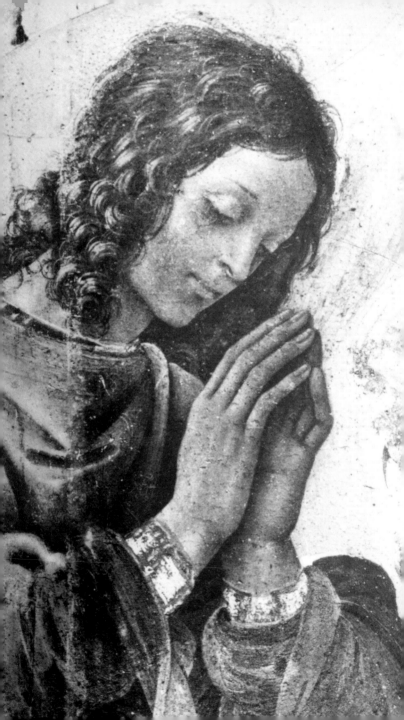

Thine is the Sole Life   O Father, with folded hands I come to offer Thee my whole being. I saturate my prayers with deep love. Give me toward Thee the simple, sincere devotion of a child.

May I intuit Thy nearness behind the words of my prayer. Teach me to feel Thee in all my emotions, to realize that Thy wisdom upholds my understanding, and to be conscious of my life as an expression of Thyself, the Sole Life.

The Divine Sculptor   Let every beat of my heart be a new word in my endless love lyric to Thee. May every sound from my lips carry secret vibrations of Thy voice. Let my every thought be bliss-saturated with Thy presence.

May every act of my will be impregnated with Thy divine vitality. Ornament with Thy grace my every concept, every expression, every ambition.

O Divine Sculptor, chisel Thou my life to Thy design!

God alone!   Who knows the secrets of all men, living and dead? God alone!

Who rested in the eternal void, before the atoms blinked glittering eyes and started the dance of creation? God alone!

We came here from some mysterious realm, we know not whence; we shall soon depart for another sphere, we know not whither. Who can explain the reason for our compulsory journeys? God alone!

With cause-effect threads we weave our intricate life patterns. Individuality and free will mark the myriad designs. Who sees their hidden harmony with a divine schema? Who unifies the bewildering variety of man's creative expression? God alone!

Who understands the origin and destination of the grand procession of living creatures that endlessly emerges from mystic chambers of space? Who can tell in what skyey mansions now dwell the countless visitors to this planet who, at the touch of Death's magic wand, instantly vanished? God alone!

Our dear ones promise to love us forever; yet when they sink into the Great Sleep, their earth memories forsaken, what value their vows? Who, without telling us in words, loves us everlastingly? who remembers us when all others forget us? who will still be with us when we leave the friends of this world? God alone!

Man plays his part, then hides behind the scenes at death, returning here in a new costume of flesh to perform again on the stage of time. Who recalls the previous roles of all persons? who is aware of their future assignments? who leads them surely through the baffling windings in the curious labyrinth of their many incarnations? God alone!

Why He is playing this game, and why He keeps the knowledge to Himself, sharing it only meagerly with us, His children, is a mystery understood by God alone.

When we dispel the delusion of physical-body identity we solve the riddle of life that sphinxlike confronts us. Who will then give us the clue to the Final Conundrum of the Cosmos? God alone!

**Tell me
Thou hast
loved me
always**

No loud or whispered words of prayer shall cloak my love for Thee. In divine unspoken language will I express my heart's devotion.

Thy voice is silence; in my soul silence may I hear Thee speak.

Tell me, O Eternal Mother, that though I knew it not, Thou hast loved me always!

**O Lord, our
first duty
is to Thee**

O Spirit! teach us to consider no other duty to be more important than our sacred duty to realize Thee, since work of any kind is possible only because Thou hast given us the power for its performance.

May we love Thee above everything else, because, without the grace of Thy life, Thy love, we could not live or love at all.

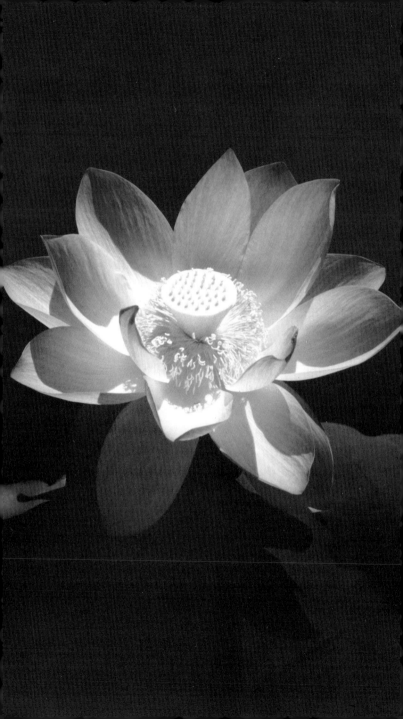

Open the petaled bars of our heart buds

Open Thou the petaled bars of our heart buds, releasing the imprisoned fragrance of love. On the winds of our spiritual perceptions the sweet odors will float to Thy secret temple.

O All-Adorable! we want our wistful breeze to blow upon Thy hidden feet.

In the nightly garden of dreams

In the nightly garden of my dreams grow many blossoms: the rarest flowers of my fancy. There, warmed by the astral dream-light, unopened buds of earthly hopes audaciously spread petals of fulfillment.

In the dream glow I spy specters of beloved forgotten faces; and sprites of dear, dead feelings, long buried in the soil of subconsciousness. All arise in shining robes. At the trumpet call of dream angels I behold the resurrection of all past experiences.

Lord, Thou hast given us freedom to forget our daily troubles by nightly visits to dreamland. May we escape from mortal sorrows forever by awakening in Thee.

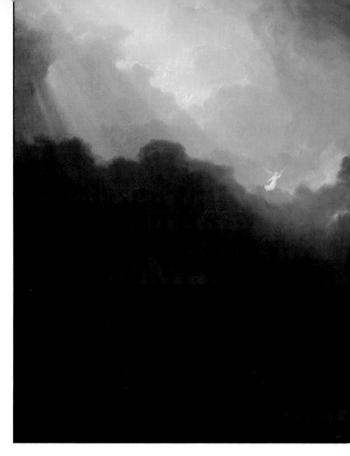

Death's reply   Thine astral airplane of earthly
parting came to take my soul
away. I wondered through what starry vaults I was
to soar, to what strange lands I was to travel.

I questioned the mystic emissary of cosmic
law. Soundlessly he answered:

"I am the pilot of ever evolving life — often
mistakenly called Terrible Death. I am thy brother,
uplifter, redeemer, friend — unloader of thy gross
burden of body troubles. I come to fetch thee away
from the valley of thy broken dreams to a won-

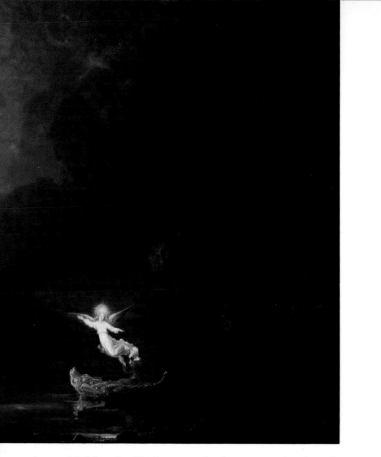

drous highland of light, to which poison vapors of sorrow cannot climb.

"I have removed thy soul bird from the cage of flesh attachment. Long imprisonment behind bars of bones madest thee used to the cage, but unwillingly; thou didst always yearn for liberty. Now, cast away fear; thou hast won thine astral freedom!

"O transitory visitor to Earth, re-enter the beauteous skies! Explore once more thine ethereal home!"

The fivefold taper of my senses

O Living Lord, help me train the truant children of my senses not to wander away from perceptions of Thee.

Direct my gaze to Thy wondrous world within, to watch Thine ever changing beauty.

May I hear the lilt of Thy secret lyre.

Teach me to feel Thy presence in me, above me, beneath me, and around me.

Bless me, that I catch the scent of Thy breath of bliss.

Let me drink forever from the sourceless river of Thine inexhaustibility.

Orientwise, with sacred rites I offer at Thine altar the candles of my senses. May their spiritualized light mingle with Thine in the first pale shaft of dawn, the brash noon brightness, the muted glow of dusk, and the night's moon silver.

O Guardian of my being, keep ever burning before Thee the fivefold taper of my love.

I am Home-ward bound at last

On the trails of time I have carelessly fallen into pits of error; but have always been rescued, O Lord, by Thine unseen hand.

I have long been fashioning an inner world of obstacles between Thee and me: shuttered huts of discouragement, barbed-wire fences of habit, stone walls of indifference, mountains of indolence, and oceans of unfaithfulness.

But now my heart is filled with divine determination, O Spirit! Should the gods promise me sextillions of years of untrammeled worldly happiness, without Self-realization, the lure would not tempt me to forsake my search for Thee.

Impediments, beware! Flee my path! I am Homeward bound.

Destroying the fortress of ignorance

Shell after shell of my yearning for Thee will break down the ramparts of delusion. With missiles of wisdom and grim guns of determination I shall destroy the fortress of my ignorance.

The devotee's aspiration
I shall be a Niagara Falls, my joy thundering in a ceaseless cascade. The powerful flood will sweep away the heavy logs of others' difficulties.

I shall be a tornado of laughter, toppling the timbers and towers of sorrow. Zooming over endless miles of mentalities, I shall demolish their troubles.

I shall be lightning flashes in the night, breathtakingly bringing to view the panorama of Thy beauty—long hidden by the darkness of unseeing eyes.

I shall be moonbeams of bliss, banishing melancholy from the earth.

I shall be rays of light, putting to flight the gloom that lurks in recesses of human thought. Through Thy grace the sudden shafts of wisdom will dispel error accumulations of countless centuries.

A prince of peace, sitting on the throne of poise
Father, teach me to be calmly active and actively calm.* May I be a prince of peace, sitting on the throne of poise and directing the kingdom of activity.

* Meditation is "active calmness." Passive calmness, as in sleep or idle daydreaming, is essentially different from active calmness—the positive state of peace found in scientific meditation. See *breath* and *Kriya Yoga* in glossary.

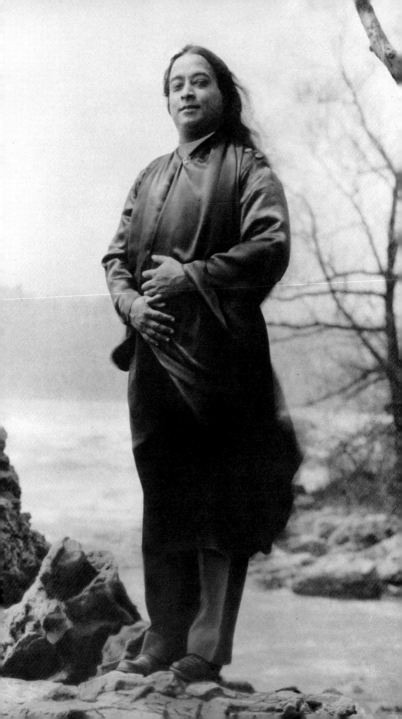

May cocktails of devotion induce God-intoxication

When Thy devotees are at prayer, from their eyes I gather rays of God-intoxication. Blending the rays into a cocktail of soul fervor, I give it to my thirsty thoughts. They drink and drink, banishing hurts and worries.

To those seeking solace I offer this magic cocktail, served in transparent glasses of my heart's goodwill and sincerity.

May drinkers of this elixir become so divinely inebriated that pain is forgotten forever.

Be Thou my Sun and Moon

Send the sunshine of Thy wisdom to guide me in my happy days of achievement; and the moon of Thy mercy when I travel in the dark nights of sorrow.

May I see goodness in others

May I never use cruel sarcasm, which, like flies, alights on the open wounds of man and thus swells his troubles.

I would emulate Thy lovable bee, attracted by the nectar of sweetness in the heart hives of others.

May I reap the harvest of Cosmic Consciousness

Once my plot of consciousness was small and devoid of all life-sustaining crops of spiritual culture.

The spring rains and the summer sunshine of Thy blessings descended on me, yet I left untilled the soil of Self-realization. Bleak winter came, shrouded in unproductivity and lost opportunities.

In anguish I cried to Thee for help. Thou didst guide me to use the best plow—the prairie breaker of Yoga*—to aid me in developing the soil of consciousness. O Supernal Sower, now Thou dost throw living seeds of Thy truth into the well-cultivated furrows of my mind.

Clearing and planting many new inner fields, I have greatly enlarged my once-tiny area of thought. I must feed innumerable families—intuitions and aspirations that ever hunger for Thee. To maintain them I constantly increase my mental holdings. In every acre I strew Thy seed whispers to me, for they yield a thousandfold.

In the short season of earthly life I aspire to reap the largest harvest—Cosmic Consciousness!

* See glossary.

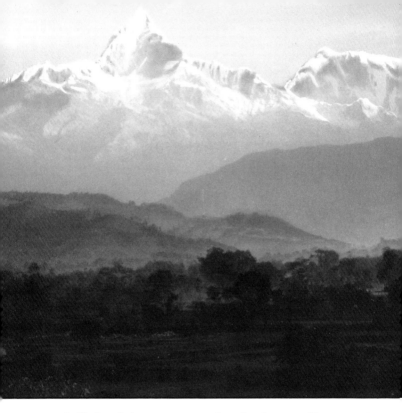

Infinitude's happy child

As Thy freeborn offspring, I want to train and use my own will; but only with Thy guidance, O Father! May all my activities lead me closer to Thy paradise of all-fulfillment.

I would be Thy happy child of Infinitude, realizing that in the divine plan Thy sons were not meant to live in a desolation of fruitless aspirations and withered hopes.

Teach me to break the shameful cords of lethargy. May I blaze my way tirelessly through the wilderness of limitations into the Fair New Land.

Thine eagle of soul progress

Make me Thine eagle of soul progress, soaring far above dusty lanes of narrowness and bigotry. Call me higher and higher, beyond earth vibrations and sun-obscuring clouds.

May I mount on the balanced wings of right living to the rarefied regions of clear perceptions of Thee. Above all storms of trials I shall climb to the heights of Thy heavenly eyrie.

Oh, make me Thine eagle of soul progress!

Thou art the highest goal of man

Can sightless men appreciate the glory of light? Can the deaf know the charms of melody? Can those blinded by self-indulgence behold the health-and-beauty rays that flow from the sun of self-control? Can bewildered ones, spiritually poor but striving only for material riches, know aught of the wealth of peace?

Father, help us to develop our powers of discrimination. May we be not satisfied with fulfillments of earthly hopes, essentially ego-tainted and limited.

O Boundless Being, Transcendent Treasure! teach us to seek the highest goal — realization of Thee.

The taper of meditation I enter the interior temple of soul research. To discover Thee I have abandoned all other duties. Darkness-haunted yet unafraid, I am groping, seeking, crying for Thee. Wilt Thou leave me alone? Reveal Thyself, O Father!

The door of memories swings open. Among the motley I look for Thee but Thou appearest not. Halt, ye throng of countless thoughts and experiences past! Come not into my sanctuary.

Firmly I close the bulging thought-pressed door and fix my mind on Thee alone.

Perceiving the astral glow of a little taper of deep concentration, I murmur a long prayer. My heart's teardrops and the gusts of my supplications almost extinguish the holy taper.

I pray no more with words but only with wistful yearning. I command my breath* to make no sound; I rebuke my boisterous love for Thee. On the cushion of peace I silently adore Thee.

The taper of meditation is burning more steadily; a divine light grows brighter and brighter. I apprehend Thy presence! Thou art I!

In joy I worship.

* See glossary.

We demand as Thy children

Father, Thou didst make us in Thine image. We pray to Thee not as beggars but as Thine offspring, co-heirs to Thy kingdom. Lovingly we demand our immortal heritage: wisdom, health, happiness, salvation, eternal joy.

Naughty or good, we are Thy children. Inspire us to seek and find Thine infallible guidance within us. May we attune our human will (that Thou gavest us to use freely) with Thy divine will.

The stricken are here at Thy door

(From a song by Ramprasad*)

The orphans and the stricken have heard of Thy grace. They are here at Thy door. Wilt Thou turn them away uncomforted?

Those whose hearts are breaking: may Thine invisible hand wipe away their scalding teardrops. Those that are lost in delusion: to whom shall they turn but to Thee?

With the dawn of Thy presence their dark troubles will take wing.

O Cosmic Mother, lift Thy veil of divine modesty and show Thy face of loving compassion.

* See glossary.

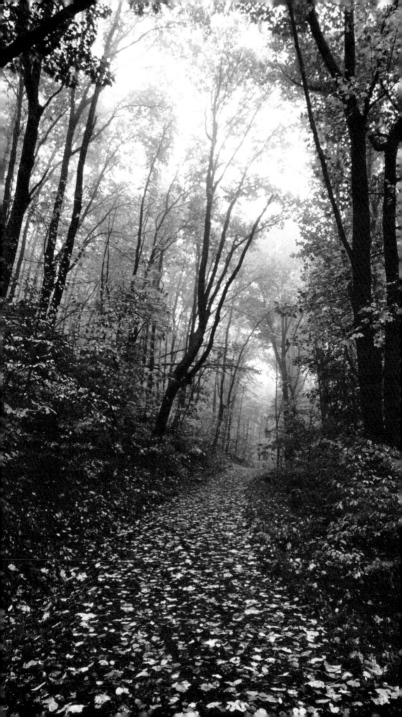

I heard Thy gentle voice saying: "Come Home"

In many lives I heard Thy gentle whisper, "Come Home," but it was drowned in the noise of unhallowed cravings.

I have forsaken the jostling crowd of desires; I would invite Thee to the virgin solitudes of my heart.

In my meditations mayest Thou banish the earth-calling lures that yet lurk in my memory. I yearn to hear again in the soul silence Thy quiet voice.

Guard me from highway robbers

O Spiritual Eye,* ever guide me, that I avoid ego detours as I travel toward the Palace of Peace.

On the winding roads of consciousness may I timely see and escape from bold highway robbers: greed, selfishness, disregard of law.

O Omniscient Light Within! show me the solutions to all problems of life.

May I overcome fear

O Divine Lion of Courage! teach me to overcome fear by understanding its uselessness. May I not anesthetize with forebodings my unlimited ability as Thy child to meet successfully any test of life.

Free me from paralyzing dreads. May I not visualize accidents and calamities, lest by the power of thought I invite them to externalize themselves.

Inspire me to put my trust in Thee, not in human precautions only. I can pass safely where bullets fly or dread bacteria abound if I realize Thou art ever with me.

May I never tremble at the thought of death. Help me to remember that for this body the Summoner shall arrive only once; and that, through his mercy, when my time is come I shall not know of it nor care.

Teach me, O Infinite Spirit! that whether I am awake or asleep, alert or daydreaming, living or dying, Thine all-protecting presence encircles me.

May I be cheerfully busy

Thou art ever at work and yet eternally smiling through countless joyous hearts. Bless me, that while I labor in the factory of life I wear, like Thee, an unfading smile.

May the waves of Thy power ever dance on the river of my daily activities.

Divine Mother, as Thou findest delight in fashioning atoms, flowers, and universes, so teach me the secret of being creatively and cheerfully busy.

I was shipwrecked on the ocean of life

My comfortable boat of earthly happiness foundered; I was shipwrecked on the ocean of life. I struggled amid the dreary waters of deceptive worldly dreams.

Sent by the winds of Thy mercy, a little raft of spiritual hope floated near me. I grasped it—I held fast! Little by little I moved onward and reached a spacious island of infinite charm.

Nymphs of Thy blessings silently gathered to take me to Thee. In Thy safe presence all hurt from my hardships vanished.

Thou lookest for my coming

O Divine Refuge! I am swimming in the sea of life, buffeted by winds of severe trials. Whether floating briefly on the crests of pleasure waves or sinking now and then into pain depths, I yearn to escape duality* by reaching Thy transcendent shores.

With every powerful stroke of my prayer I am moving nearer to Thee. I shall never give up, for I know Thou dost eagerly look for my coming.

***Aum*, the heartbeat of creation**

O Cosmic Vibration, manifest Thyself to me as the voice of Infinity. May I intuit the Christ Consciousness† in Thee.

O Omnipresent Sound of *Aum, Amen*! Reverberate through me, expanding my mind from the body to the universe. Teach me to feel in Thee the immortal heartbeat of creation.

* See *maya* in glossary.
† See *Sat-Tat-Aum* and *Aum* in glossary.

**I come with
the myrrh
of reverence**

I come to Thee with folded hands, bowed head, and heart laden with the myrrh of reverence.

From the hearts of all Thine other lovers I have distilled a fragrant essence of devotion and mixed the drops with my tears. In those sacred waters may I bathe Thy lotus feet.

Thou art my Parents; I am Thy child. Thou art the Master; I will obey the silent command of Thy voice.

**Thou art my
Protector**

May I not rouse the fiery tempers of undisciplined natures; but if I become their target I shall silently hide behind Thy rock of refuge in my soul.

O Divine Protector! without Thee I am unsafe in even the most unassailable earthly fort. Be Thou my impenetrable shield against the exploding shells of trials.

Bless me, that with divine surgery I heal all who suffer from the shrapnel wounds of life.

Give us a true conception of brotherhood
Divine Mother, give us a new, true conception of brotherhood. May we forsake wars and heal the wounds of all nations with the salve of Christ-love and the lasting balm of sympathetic understanding.

Cosmic Mother, awaken in us Thine impartial love for all; bless us that we be free from the sway of greed and delusion. Inspire us to build a new world—one in which famine, disease, and ignorance will be only memories of a dismal past.

Creative Mother, arouse us to knowledge of Thy plan, when Thou didst form the cosmos and people it with rational creatures. Let us be ashamed to act like savage animals, devoid of reason, settling their differences only by might. Help us to solve all problems not by jungle logic but by reason and unfaltering trust in Thee.

O Mother of All, teach us to call each man by his rightful name of Brother.

Thought at Christmas
Beneath the Christmas tree of civilization, with its many branches of races, may we lay imperishable presents of goodwill, spiritual service, and unconditional love for all. These are the gifts that Christ wants to receive.

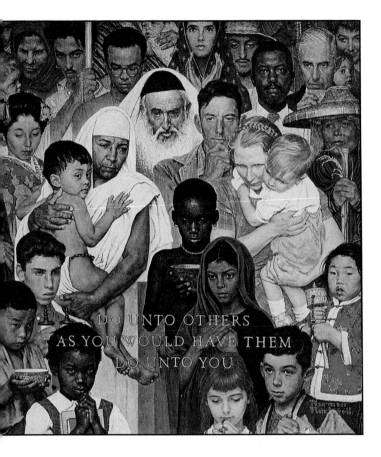

The Lord's Prayer: *
a humble interpretation

O Heavenly Father, Mother, Friend, Beloved God! may our ceaseless silent utterance of Thy holy Name transform us to Thy likeness.

Inspire us, that our matter worship be changed to adoration of Thee. Through our purified hearts may Thy perfect kingdom come on earth, and all nations be liberated from misery. Let the soul freedom within us be manifested outwardly.

May our wills grow strong in overcoming worldly desires and finally be attuned to Thy faultless will.

Give us our daily bread: food, health, and prosperity for the body; efficiency for the mind; and, above all, Thy love and wisdom for the soul.

It is Thy law that "with the same measure ye mete, it shall be measured to you."† May we forgive those who offend us, ever mindful of our own need for Thine unmerited mercy.

Leave us not in the pit of temptations into which we have fallen through our misuse of Thy gift of reason. Shouldst Thou wish to test us, O

* Matthew 6:9-13 and Luke 11:24.
† Luke 6:38.

Spirit, may we realize Thou art enchanting beyond any earthly temptation.

Help us to deliver ourselves from the shadowy bonds of the sole evil: ignorance of Thee.

For Thine is the kingdom, and the power, and the glory, forever. *Amen.*

May I drown in Thine Ocean and live

I come to Thee with my song of gladness. Treasures from the secret safe of my soul I bring eagerly to Thee. I gather for Thee the devotion honey in the hive of my heart. All that is mine is Thine.

I was parched in the desert of false hopes. Now my desires have slaked their thirst forever, drinking of Thee.

Whiffs from Thy sweet-scented flame are floating to me. My taper of happiness is set ablaze by sparks from Thy fire of bliss.

I was dying amidst the mirage oases of earth. Now the joyous waves of Thy Spirit engulf me. May I drown in Thine Ocean and live!

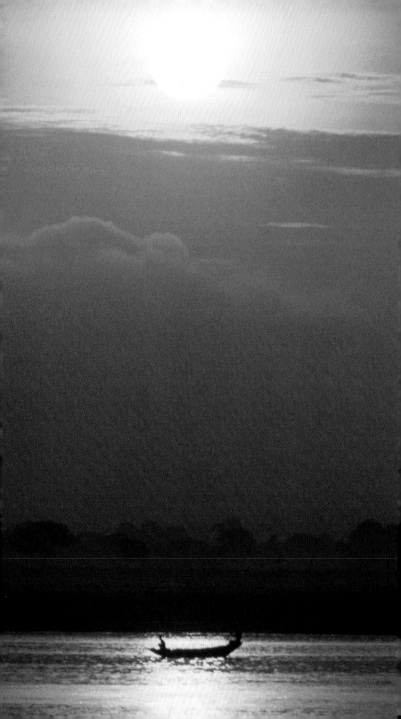

**Our purified
rivers reach
Thy Sea**

O Oceanic Being, guide Thou the rivulets of our joys, that they be not lost in the sands of shortlived sense satisfactions.

May the brooklets of our sympathies not end in the desert of dreary selfishness.

Let the little, lonely, separately moving streamlets of our affections merge in Thy lake of illimitable love.

May the narrow rivers of our lives be widened by torrential rains of Thy blessings, and pass through vast lowlands of humbleness, self-sacrifice, and consideration for others, to enter in purity Thy Blissful Sea.

**Remove Thou
the veils
of creation**

O Lord, the veils of matter conceal Thee from me. How long wilt Thou remain invisible behind the lovely screens of lilies and roses, the clouds of burning gold, and the silent star-decked night? Though they hide Thee, I love them because they hint at Thy presence. Yet I yearn to see Thee as Thou truly art, Thy robes of creation laid aside.*

---

* See *Sat-Tat-Aum* in glossary.

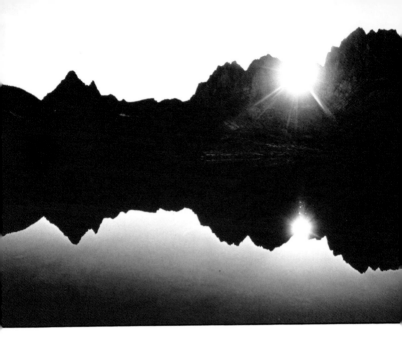

May I still the gale of passions

O Spirit, may I find Thee in meditation by banishing restlessness, sensory impressions, and consciousness of breath. *

Let the gale of passions and desires be stilled by a magic wand of divine perceptions.

In a rippleless mental lake may I behold the undistorted reflection of the moon of my soul, glistening with the light of Thy presence.

* See glossary.

Glance Thou into my ardent eyes

Make me transparent with purity, that I manifest Thy healing light within me.

Still the restlessly moving mirror of my mind, that it reflect only Thine infinite face.

Fling wide the windows of faith, that I inhale Thy fragrance of peace.

O Self-Illumined, O Ineffable Effulgence, glance Thou into my ardent eyes, that I be blind forever to all but Thee.

Each of us reflects Thine individuality

O Sun of Life, as Thou didst first peep into mortal cups of mind, filled with the molten liquid of Thy vitality, Thou wert caught within the microcosm of human feelings.

From Thy gaze each of Thy children retained a unique facet of Thine individuality. In their lives I behold expressions of Thine inexhaustible variety.

I am a spark of Thy cosmic fire

When the sparks of creation first flew from Thy bosom of flame, I sang in the chorus of astral lights that heralded the coming of the worlds.* I am an immortal spark of Thy cosmic fire.

May I help, not punish, wrongdoers

O Father of All, may I feel that even he who does me mortal injury is my brother, made in Thine image, and existing only temporarily in darkness. Banish from my mind the vengeful "tit-for-tat" spirit.

Let my sympathy go out to all, including those whom society, to protect itself, has imprisoned. Teach me to desire eagerly their redemption and solace in Thee.

May I not increase the ignorance of wrongdoers by my intolerance or vindictiveness. Inspire me to help them by my forgiveness, prayers, and tears of gentle love.

* "I was set up from everlasting, from the beginning, or ever the earth was."—Proverbs 8:23.

Make me a smile millionaire

O Silent Laughter of Spirit! smile Thou through my soul. Let my soul smile through my heart, and my heart smile through my eyes.

Make me a smile millionaire, that I may freely scatter to poor hearts the riches of Thy smiles.

Enthrone Thyself in the castle of my countenance, O Prince of Smiles! No rebels of hypocrisy shall enter; Thou wilt be protected by my unassailable sincerity.

Thou art the Sole Doer

Thou art walking through my feet, wielding my arms of activity, throbbing in my heart, flowing through my breath, and weaving thoughts in my brain. It is Thy meteoric will that courses daily through the skies of my human will.

Let me feel it is Thou that hast become I. Oh, make me Thyself, that I behold the little bubble of me, floating in Thee!

Be Thou President of a United World

Divine Creator, President of the Universe, Chief Executive of Planets, Stars, and Galaxies! Thy democratic rule, giving the rights of free will and self-evolution to Thy citizen children, is bringing them nearer and nearer to Thine ideals.

Created with the consciousness of omnipresence, we had from Thee a birthright of eternal freedom. Alas, we imprisoned our universality behind bars of selfish interests and narrowheartedness. May we learn to express our soul warmth of love and understanding, melting all icy boundaries of exclusiveness.

Bless us, O Father, that we form a United World, electing Thee as our Perpetual Spiritual President. With Thy guidance, may we govern ourselves rightly through conscience and soul discrimination.

Teach us to enrich our spiritual opportunities and sympathies by enlarging the circle of our patriotic love, including in it all inhabitants of the earth, regardless of color, caste, class, sex, or creed.

O Cosmic Lord, help us to respect, with kindness, the independence of all Thy freeborn sons. Whether they are good or temporarily error-intoxicated, may we honor all as Thy children.

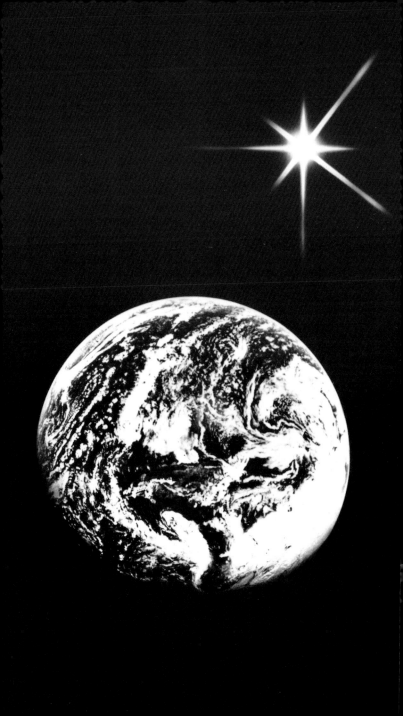

Prayer at dawn

At dawn and the opening of lotus buds, my soul flower softly unfolds to receive Thy light. Each petal is bathed in rays of bliss. The early breezes waft the perfume of Thy presence.

Bless me, that with the spreading aurora I spread to all men Thy message of love. With the awakening day may I awaken countless souls with my own and bring them to Thee.

Prayer at noon

The sun is at zenith; Thine outer world is filled with vigor. Express through me Thy vitality and creativeness.

O Invisible Lord, Thy presence permeates the sunrays. They recharge my body battery, that I be strong and tireless. In the heat of the day's activities I drink from Thy fountain of joy.

Thine infinite beams shine on all places, crowded or empty. As I walk the populous and the lonely paths of life, may I, too, radiate unchangeably the light of Thy love.

Prayer at eventide   The day is done. Purified by its sunshine, I pass through the faintly starlit portals of evening. I bow to Thine approaching Spirit of calmness.

What prayers shall I offer? for I have no words worthy of Thee. On the altar of my heart I will light a fire of devotion. Shall that little blaze suffice to attract Thee to my temple — dimly illumined, long dark with ignorance?

Come, O Lord, I yearn for Thee!

Prayer at night   In the peace of night I worship Thee. The sunlight that revealed a myriad earthly allurements has vanished.

One by one I shut the doors of my senses, lest the fragrance of the rose or the song of the nightingale distract my love from Thee.

Like Night, I adore Thee in hiddenness and silence. Within the shrine of darkness I invoke Thee, Blessed and Beloved! *

* Earlier versions of the prayers at dawn, noon, eventide, and night are available on recordings by Paramahansa Yogananda. See page 203. *(Publisher's Note)*.

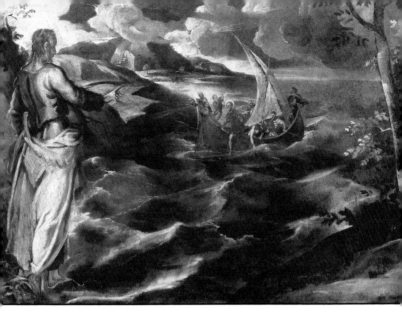

May I calm the storms of restless desires

With the power that flows from perceptions of Thee, may I calm by Christlike command[*] my storms of restless desires.

Blessed Spirit, help me to subdue the incessant ripples of the little wave of my life, that Thine oceanic vastness spread over me.

In the limpid waters of my soul let me behold the unruffled reflection of Thy face of stillness.

[*] "And he arose, and rebuked the wind, and said unto the sea, Peace, be still. And the wind ceased, and there was a great calm."—Mark 4:39.

Right thinking for prosperity Thou art my Father, I am Thine offspring. Thou art Spirit; I am made in Thine image. Thou art Creator and Owner of the universe. Good or naughty, I am Thy child, with the right to command the cosmos.

I have been truant and wandered away from my Home of cosmic plenty. Help me to reidentify my mind with Thine. Expand me; let me feel again I am like unto Thee.

Rescue my mind, shipwrecked through thoughts of error and now confined to a tiny isle of consciousnesss.

By Thy grace I shall rediscover my true nature, that of omnipresent Spirit, and have dominion* over the world of matter.

Be thou my Beacon of Wisdom If, driven by squalls of ignorance, my mind raft nears the dangerous rocks of insatiable desires, mayest Thou warn me, O Beacon of Wisdom! I am ever seeking the safe shores of righteousness.

---

* "And God said, Let us make man in our image, after our likeness: and let them have dominion over…all the earth."
—Genesis 1:26.

By trials may I perfect myself

O Lord of Law, may I wear my scars of trials like deserved medals of chastisement, presented to me by the sacred hands of Thy perfect Justice.

Let my daily difficulties act as antidotes against delusion and rid me of false hopes of worldly happiness.

May the tears that flow from me at others' cruel actions wash away from my mind some hidden taint.

Let each sharp stroke of the pickax of unpleasantness expose within me new wisdom depths.

May the unhallowed darkness of ordinary existence so frighten me that I rushingly seek Thy realm of purity and light.

Let life's sudden sword thrusts force from me only a cry for Thy succor.

May the hurtful diggings of circumstance into the soil of my being uncover the ever bubbling well-spring of Thy solace.

Let the ugliness of unkindness in others impel me to make myself beautiful with loving-kindness.

May harsh speech from my companions remind me to use sweet words always.

If stones from evil minds are cast at me, let me send in return only missiles of goodwill.

As a jasmine vine sheds its flowers over the hands delivering ax blows at its roots, so, on all who act inimically toward me may I shower the blossoms of forgiveness.

May I find my Self in all   Teach me to feel that, but for the right use of Thy grace and wisdom, I might have been lame, leprous, or blind. Even though I deserved such a fate, I would earnestly crave to be healed.

O Divine Mother, whenever I see men maimed in limb or shattered by sorrow, may I feel that it is Thine omnipresent Spirit suffering in those forms. Teach me to sympathize with all my brothers and to fight to free them from miseries, even as I would try to free myself.

Craving, struggling, weeping, and smiling for others, at last may I find my Self in all.

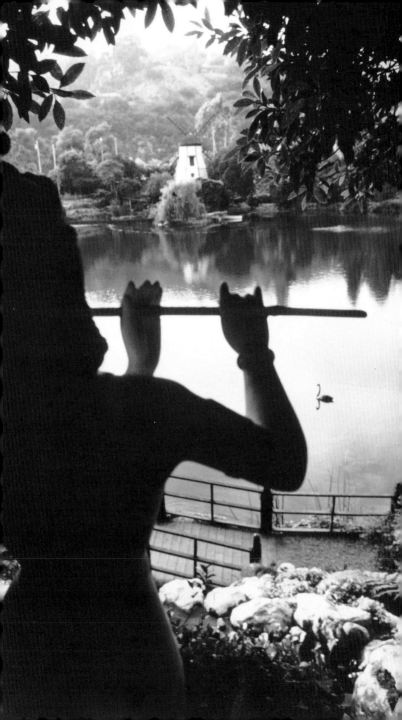

Thy magnum opus of *Aum*   O Master Piper, blow through the flutes of all religions Thine entrancing song of Oneness. Ornament the theme with grace notes from the richness of Thy Spirit.

By attunement with Thee may we bring our hearts' fragmentary melodies to divine completion.

Teach us to hear the perfect music: Thy magnum opus of *Aum*.*

Heavenly Thief of Hearts   The rays of joy spreading in the firmament of my inner silence are promises of Thine approach. Whether Thou deignest to appear soon or late, some day I shall seize Thee, O Heavenly Thief of Hearts!

Meditation and devotion   O Spirit, teach me to pray with deep concentration, and to imbue scientific meditation with devotion. May my heart daily become more pure by all-surrendering love for Thee.

* See glossary.

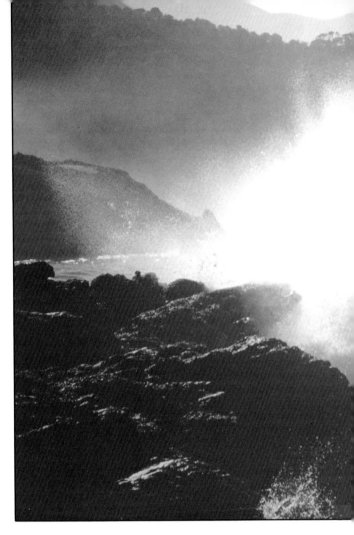

I am a wave of joy

I am sea foam spumed from the deeps of joy. I am a wave of joy, seeking to dance in all billows of joy, struggling to be the ocean of joy. May the ripples of my laughter spread endlessly, finally subsiding on the bosom of infinite joy.

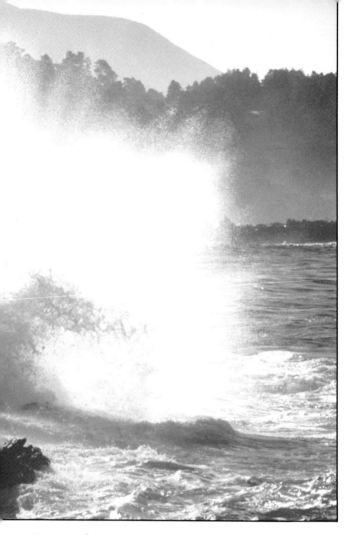

Boom Thou on the shores of my mind

O Holy Vibration of *Aum*,[*] boom Thou on my inner shores. Destroy the boundary thoughts of flesh confinement.

In meditation let me hear Thy subtle ocean-like reverberation in my body, mind, and soul;

[*] See glossary.

and in my environment of creation: first in my immediate surroundings, then spreading to all towns, cities, the earth, the solar system, and the universe.

May I be conscious of my augmented being in the vast cosmic body of Nature.

For Thee: a bouquet of all loves Our love for others is possible only because we have received from Thee the power to feel affection; inspire us, therefore, to offer Thee our supreme love.

Thou hast given us parents, brothers, sisters, cousins, marriage partner, children, and friends, that we learn to love Thee with the varied expressions and natural nuances of all types of relationships.

O Eternal Lover, O Kingly Kinsman! teach me to make a bouquet of all the flowers of my human loves and to lay it on Thine altar.

If, because of my confusion of loyalties, I cannot now present to Thee a full bouquet, I shall pluck one blossom, the rarest of all, and offer it at Thy feet. Wilt Thou receive it?

May I abandon the anger habit

O Eternal Tranquillity! save me from attacks of fury fever that shock my nerves and inflame my brain.

May I abandon the anger habit that brings unhappiness to me and my companions. Let me not indulge in fits of selfish vexation that alienate from me the affection of my loved ones.

May I never invigorate my resentments by attentively refueling their fires.

O Queen of Quietude! whenever I am rageful place Thou before me a chastening mirror in which to see myself made ugly by passion. Let me not appear disfigured before others, my face wrath-wrecked.

I would solve the difficulties of life through thoughts and acts of love, not of hate. Bless me, that I heal anger hurts in myself with the salve of self-respect, and anger hurts in others with the balsam of kindness.

May I realize, O Spirit, that even my worst enemy is still my brother; and that, even as Thou lovest me, Thou lovest him.

I fly from life to life With living threads of Thy beauty my winsome wings were woven. Endowed with a spark of immortality, I have flown from life to life.

I escape from all who audaciously try to possess me; I belong only to Thee. No transiency enthralls me; my true Home is Thy Changeless Spirit.

Thou hast clothed barren eternity in the verdure of multicolored cycles. In the forest of incarnations I flit gaily from tree to tree. I shall alight at last, O Lord, upon Thine outstretched hand.

May I savor with Thy zest all innocent pleasures Divine Mother, teach me to live with delight. May I enjoy my earthly duties and the countless beauties of creation. Help me to train my senses to observe and appreciate Thy wondrous world of Nature.

Let me savor with Thy zest all innocent pleasures. Save me from negation and unwarranted kill-joy attitudes.

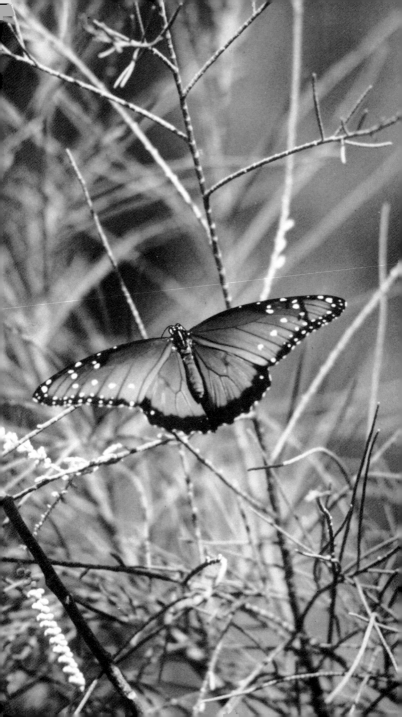

We are Thy burned children, wailing for Thy help

The fascinating fire of wrong pleasures attracts Thy children. The silent voice of conscience warns them of the scorching, scarring consequences; but men often blindly seize the flames of temporary exhilarations. Many plunge greedy hands into the devouring blaze and are badly injured. They wail for Thy help.

O Patient Physician, Thou art always near with the unguent of forgiveness and love. Teach us to heed Thine inward admonitions, that we give to Thee gladsome songs, instead of helpless cries as we writhe in unnecessary pain.

We are Thy heedless children, and the fiery excitements of the world allure us. Teach us to play only with the searless flames of Thy Spirit.

Unbroken oneness

Teach me, O Father, to find my oneness with Thee in the peace within and the tumult without. I care not whether silence or noise surround me, if at all times and in all places I may feel Thine enveloping presence.

**Prayer of
my heart**
Make my soul Thy temple!
Make my heart Thine altar!
Make my love Thy home!

May Thy love shine forever on the sanctuary of my devotion, and may I be able to awaken Thy love in all hearts.

**The gaze
of truth**
My human eyes are enthralled, O Lord, with the changeful panorama of life and the gay prodigality of Nature — the multicolored flowers and the silent sailing clouds.

Open in me the divine eye* that beholds in all beauty only Thy sovereign beauty. With the gaze of truth may I perceive in the universe nothing but Thee.

* See *spiritual eye* in glossary.

**May I
discipline
the senses**
Train me to be vigilant, lest the senses don stolen royal trappings and the mirage cloak of happiness, and, so disguised, deceive me while they desecrate my bodily temple.

Help me to discipline my unwise, wayward senses, that they spiritualize their desires.

The gaudy sirens of the senses offer earthly pleasures. Thou hast arrayed Thine angel joys in robes of simplicity; may I follow them to the Eternal Eden.

**Thou art hiding behind
a veil of
cosmic rays**
O Light of Supernatural Subtlety! Thou dost hide behind Thine ultraviolet rays in the sun and in earth-bombarding cosmic rays.

Lord, Thine etheric veil, patterned with intricate crisscrosses of countless invisible currents, effectively conceals Thee from me. Drop Thou the raiment of space, that I see Thee without matter illusions.

Save us from the dragnet of delusion By stealth the fisherman, Transitoriness, deludes us. We swim in the shallow waters of false assurances of safety, the while a deadly net of ignorance is closing in upon us. In the daily haul, many men are caught—few escape.

O Measureless Mercy, save us from the dread dragnet of desires and matter attachment! May we dive into silent deep-sea spaces of divine communion and become uncapturable.

Diving for the Pearl of Great Price O Fathomless Ocean of Treasure! may I dive deep in seas of meditation for Thy wisdom pearls.

Teach me to plunge with headlong faith, carrying the sharp dagger of conscience to protect me against sharks of passions.

If I fail in one or many searches, let me not believe the vast inner main devoid of riches; rather, may I find fault with myself for doubts and unmethodical diving.

By my sacred perseverance, guide me to discover in the most secret waters of consciousness the Pearl of Great Price.

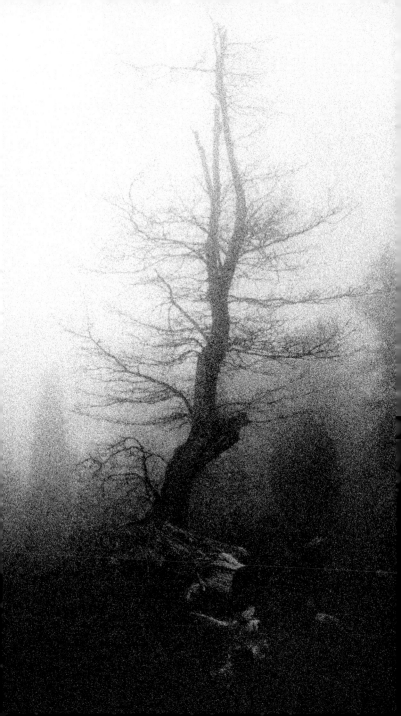

May my gratitude be changeless

When the summer of good fortune warms my tree of life, it easily burgeons with fragrant blossoms of thankfulness.

During winter months of misfortune, O Lord, may my denuded branches changelessly waft toward Thee a secret scent of gratitude.

I will be Thine always

I may go far, beyond the uttermost star, but I will be Thine always.

Devotees may come, devotees may go; but I will be Thine always.

I may bound over the billows of many incarnations, forlorn beneath skies of loneliness; but I will be Thine always.

The world, engrossed in Thy playthings, may forsake Thee; but I will be Thine always.

My voice may become feeble and fail me; yet with the voice of my soul I shall whisper: "I will be Thine always."

Trials, disease, and death may riddle and rend me. While the embers of my memory still flicker, look Thou into my dying eyes; they shall mutely say: "I will be Thine always."

Heal us in body, mind, and soul   O Spirit, teach us to heal the body by recharging it with Thy cosmic energy, to heal the mind by concentration and cheerfulness, and to heal the disease of soul ignorance by the divine medicine of meditation on Thee.

Healing affirmation   O Divine Spirit, Thou didst create my body. It is well, for Thou art present in it. Thy Being is perfect. I am made in Thine image: I am perfect.

Affirmation for healing others   You are a child of the Heavenly Father. His immortal life energy pervades all your body cells. Your whole being is vibrant with His presence: you are well.

Dewdrops of repentance

In the garden of soul awakening the dewdrops of my repentance gathered at Thy lotus feet.

By those tears, precious to Thee, my heart was fully cleansed.

O Virtue! thou art infinitely more charming than Vice

Teach us, O Spirit, to regard virtue not with dread but with love. May we realize that obedience to the rules of Thine ethical code will crown us with the laurel of Thy grace.

Thou hast issued the commandments of righteousness to safeguard our happiness. May we shun the path of wrongdoing, which always leads to suffering. Let us see that virtue is infinitely more charming than vice.

Help us to understand that evil, which at first may seem delightful, gradually acts as poison; and that good, in the beginning often bitter to our taste, eventually becomes nectar-sweet.

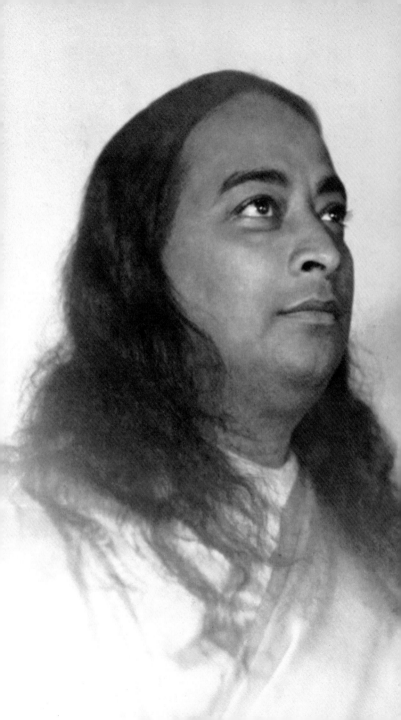

The sun gaze of my love ne'er sets

I take a sacred vow: Never shall the sun gaze of my love sink below the horizon of my thought of Thee. Never will I lower the vision of my lifted eyes to place it on aught but Thee.

Never will I do anything that reminds me not of Thee. Actions springing from ignorance lead to nightmares. May I weave only sweet dreams of noble achievements, for they are Thy dreams.

Blow through the flute of my being

Loving Lord, with my hands help Thy children; speak Thou through my voice; use my mind to inspire others.

Breathe with my breath; for through the fragile flute of my being Thou alone canst blow the eternals of Thy song.

* See glossary.

All creation is Thine inimitable handiwork
Teach us to love the birds and beasts; and the frail wayside flowers and mute grasses, oft crushed by our unheeding feet.

The countless forms in Nature are expressions of Thy versatile genius—originals from Thy ceaselessly vibrating fingers. May we see in all creation Thine inimitable handiwork.

Heavenly Hart, I hunted Thee in the forest of consciousness
Clad in the hunter's green of selfish desires, I pursued Thee in the forest of consciousness, O Divine Hart! The sound of my loud prayers startled Thee; Thou didst swiftly flee. I raced after Thee; but my erratic chase, the hue and cry of restlessness, caused Thee to retreat still farther.

Stealthily I crept toward Thee with my spear of concentration, but my aim was unsteady. As Thou didst bound away I heard in secret echoes of Thy footfalls: "Without devotion thou art a poor, poor marksman!"

Even when I held firmly my meditation missile, Thine echo resounded: "I am beyond thy mental dart; I am beyond!"

At last, in submissive wisdom I entered the silent cave of selfless love. Lo! Thou, the Hart of Heaven, camest willingly within.

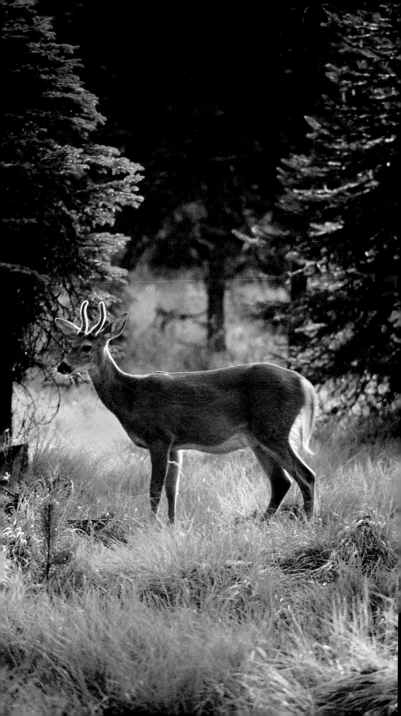

We are actors in Thy cosmic pictures

Thy kaleidoscopic sound-picture, the ever changing drama of turbulence and calm, is only a vast structure of illusion.

Our dreams of birth and death, of contrasts and paradoxes, of comedies and tragedies are nought but talking pictures, produced to instruct and entertain.

O Lord of Phantasmagoria, through Thy cosmic vibratory current of *Aum** Thou art daily showing us, on the screen of our consciousness, a new chapter of scenes in the infinite serial of Thy shadow show.

Each of us plays parts of both joy and sorrow in Thy "supertalkies." May we play them well. Give us respite now and then, that we retire among our thought audiences in a balcony of introspection, there to behold with serene detachment the re-enacting of our roles.

May we view the adverse episodes in our lives with the eye of wisdom, saying: "Ah, that was a good film, full of life and worthwhile struggle. I learned much from it."

* See glossary.

Prayer for peace
(Written in 1944)

Father, all peoples are weary of the carnage, the loss of throbbing lives (O Youth, so dead, so deathless!) and of man's material heritage (O Monte Cassino, symbol of centuried dignity, destroyed in a day!).*

We learn hardly that war, like crime, does not pay. Solving nothing, World War I led only to World War II. Victor and vanquished alike still see but afar the goal of virtue and brotherhood.

Thou alone art almighty, O Father; listen to our supplications and swiftly terminate the war in justice. Help to end the bombings of the innocent young and the helpless old. May our prayers and Thy blessings mitigate the war-creating karma of nations, and quickly stop this affrighting bloodshed.

Divine Majesty, Thou art sitting on the throne of all hearts. Inspire us with spiritual understanding that we overcome fear and hate. With faith in Thee, may we be steadfast in the path of righteousness.

O Lord of Law! teach us to remove the true cause of war—heedlessness of Thy word.

* This ancient monastery in Italy was demolished by bombing on February 15, 1944.

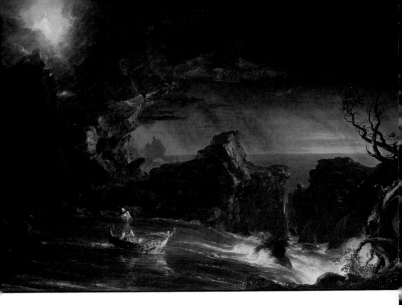

Master Mariner, take charge of my boat

O Father, my little raft of meditation is buffeting furious storms of distraction. On this boisterous mental sea I am yet heading toward Thy shores. Master Mariner, come, take charge of my boat!

I am immortal Spirit

O Omnipresent Protector! when clouds of war send rains of gas and fire, be Thou my bomb shelter.

In life and death, in disease, famine, pestilence, or poverty may I ever cling to Thee. Help me to realize I am immortal Spirit, untouched by the changes of childhood, youth, age, and world upheavals.

Save me from wrong beliefs   I am lost in the wastelands of wrong beliefs; I cannot find my way. O Compassionate Lord, lead me to Thyself, who art my Home!

I valiantly struggle toward Thee   O Eternal Polaris! where'er I roam, the magnetic needle of my mind compass ever and ever points to Thee.

Buffeted by gusts of chance or drenched by rains of misfortune, I nevertheless direct my mind to look always toward Thee.

The dove of my love, winging through clouds of bewilderments, storms of distractions, and whirlwinds of destiny, yet will infallibly discover the way to Thee.

My taper of remembrance of Thee   I may lose my way and roam in darkness, but, O Divine Mother! see that the tiny taper of my remembrance of Thee be never extinguished by gusts of disbelief.

I sought all earthly things, finally to discover that I crave only Thee. Come, be with me always!

Repair my nerve wires, O Mystic Electrician!

Come Thou, O Mystic Electrician! My little soul cottage by the brook of life is in need of repairs.

The nerve wiring has been shaken and torn by the winds of the years. The multihued lamps of my senses are no longer effulgent.

O Builder of Bodies, O Divine Dynamo of all cosmic currents of life force! resurrect the deadened wires of my wrecked nerves and infuse them with Thy power, that my senses gleam again with Thy glory.

I am the bulb and Thou art the Light within it. The truth and the miracle is this:

Thou art the Bulb and the Light.

Forget me not, though I forget Thee

O Father, from the garden of the dawn I pluck blossoms of light as offerings at Thy feet.

May the shooting star of my love gloriously race across the dark skies of my long obliviousness of Thee.

Forget me not, though I forget Thee. Remember me, though I remember Thee not.

Purify me in a furnace of trials

The ore of my life is smelting in a furnace of trials. All baseness is being scorified in the fires of experience and sacred aspirations.

O Divine Artisan, reduce to dross my weaknesses! Harden me into the tempered steel of fortitude and soul strength. Help me to fashion my purified metal into effective weapons of right tenacity and self-control. With the sword of mind equilibrium may I rout inner enemies that would distract me from the sole thought of Thee.

From joy I came, for joy I live

From joy I came, for joy I live, and in Thy sacred joy I shall melt again.

Teach me to find my joy not in the world but in Thee. Discovering Thy presence in the joy born of meditation and good actions, I shall feel no need for pleasures born of the misguided senses.

O Father, Thou art ever new Joy; Thou art the lasting Joy of the soul; Thou art the Joy that I seek.

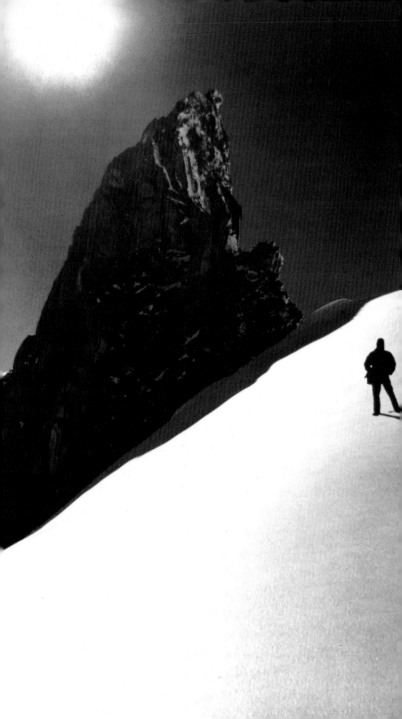

Prayer to the Holy Trinity

O Triune Lord! Beatific Trinity, Irresolvable Unity, *Sat-Tat-Aum* — God the Father, transcending creation; God the Son, the guiding Christ Consciousness immanent in creation; and God the Holy Ghost, the secret Vibration of *Aum* that externalizes all creation!* Lead me to the final Wisdom, the ultimate Truth.†

Guide my tireless efforts to attain perfect knowledge of Thy Law. May I succeed in climbing the sacred mountain of Self-realization and stand at last on the shining summit, face to face with Thee, O Inconceivable Spirit Divine!

Spiritualize us, O Infinite Alchemist!

O Infinite Alchemist, spiritualize us! Turn our weakness into strength, our wrong thoughts into truth perceptions.

Transform our ugly demons of selfish ambitions into fairies of soaring aspirations; our painful ignorance into blissful wisdom; and our base ores of inertia into the purified gold of spiritual accomplishments.

* See *Sat-Tat-Aum* in glossary.
† "God is a Spirit: and they that worship Him must worship Him in Spirit and in Truth."—John 4:24.

I am Thy divine dewdrop

I am Thy dewdrop, quivering on the leaf of life-and-death that floats on Thy shoreless sea.

I am Thy truant dewdrop, returning at last to the Hallowed Home.

I am Thine immortal dewdrop, dancing on the petals of past-present-future.

I am Thy love-enchanted dewdrop, sliding safely over the leaf of earthly lures to enter Thy taintless waters of wisdom. I want not to lose myself but to become infinitely enlarged by merging in Thy Sea.

I shall be Thine omnipresent dewdrop, imbibed by all God-thirsty lips.

All power is divine

Thou art the mysterious Electricity of my body, moving the intricate mechanism of flesh, bones, muscles, and nerves. Thy life force is present in my every breath and heartbeat.

O Sole Doer in Man and the Universe! may I realize that all power is divine and flows only from Thee.

May I live less by food and more by cosmic light

O Divine Life Energy that directly sustainest my body! Thou dost convert and spiritualize my food — solids, liquids, and air — into Thy revivifying rays. Teach me, O Spirit, to live less and less by gross matter and more and more by cosmic light.

Thy power is present in my body bulb. I recharge myself with Thine omnipresent life.

Correct my defective vision

I have long been suffering from the jaundiced vision of earthliness. Instead of perceiving Thee, O Ever Living Spirit, my disordered view sees only the pale corpse of matter. Wilt Thou not heal me, that with perfect wisdom sight I behold in all things Thy transfiguring presence?

Misleading folly fires	During the night of error we pursued the will-o'-the-wisp of sense happiness. Far from the paths of soul progress, we stumbled through marshes of disillusionment.

O Ever Watchful Father, let not bog-born flames of folly, the *ignes fatui* of our passions, lead us into sense quagmires.

May we, Thine eager pilgrim children, easily reach our Home by following the inner light — intuition,* Thy holy beacon.

Revive my friendship with Thee	O Patient Heart, teach me to revive by meditation my old friendship with Thee. May I realize that in my journey toward divine expansion, incarnation after incarnation Thou and Guru have been and will be my only Eternal Friends.

Be my Captain	O Heavenly Father, be Thou the Captain of the boat of my daily activities and bring it to the shores of divine fulfillment.

* See glossary.

Come, O Perfect Joy! Divine Mother, be Thou the only flame in our hearts, banishing all darkness within us. In our tears of love for Thee, wash away our love for material possessions. In the bliss of our communion with Thee, destroy forever all sorrows.

Unite our little hearts into a heart great enough to contain Thine omnipresence. In the mirror of Thy divinity may we behold ourselves as perfect. Let the fire of our love for Thee soar triumphantly above the tiny hissing flames of earthly desires.

A million distractions, disguised as Thee, constantly delude us. Come, O Perfect Joy, into the waiting temple of our devotion! Be Thou the Polestar during our wanderings in the night of ignorance, leading us safely to our haven in Thee.

Ego, the impersonator My ego* may strut in pride, saying: "I am thou!"

Ignoring the tiny boasting masquerader, I shall seek my soul Self, fragrant with countless humilities.

Ever instruct me in my identity, O Lord! May I inly hear Thy whisper: *I am thou!*

* See *egoism* in glossary.

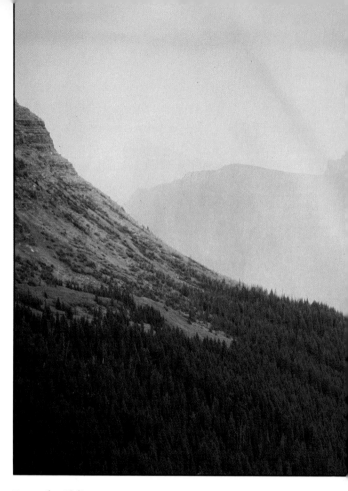

I am building a rainbow bridge to reach Thee

An age-old gulf has lain between Thee and me, ever widening with the rush of the waters of my obliviousness of Thee.

Now I stand on the rocky strand of matter and look longingly for Thy distant shores of etheric beauty.

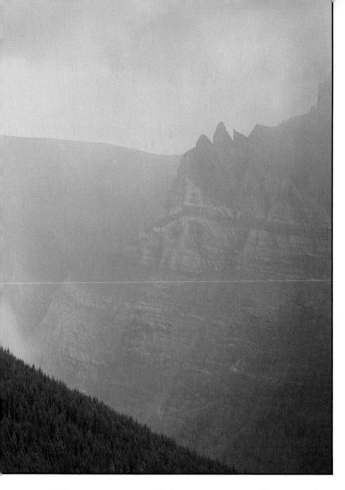

I have summoned divine inner architects that are building across the gulf a rainbow bridge of my constant remembrance of Thee. The strong girders of self-control are being riveted. Soon I shall be able to reach Thee!

Removing the debris of delusion The kingdom of my mind is begrimed with ignorance. By steady rains of diligence in self-discipline may I remove from my cities of spiritual carelessness the ancient debris of delusion.

Let the deluge wash away the disfiguring slums of narrow-mindedness and race-and-creed prejudice.

O Lord, may the soiled untidy thought children of my realm bathe in Thy waters of purity and orderliness.

I am Thy bird of paradise I am a bird of paradise, fashioned by Thee. Thou hast costumed me in grace, color, and beauty: soft down of tenderness and golden plumes of soul unfoldment.

Ever seeking the Eden of bliss, I have winged my way through life's somber skies. Streaks of dark despondency have blurred my brightness.

Come Thou, O Lord, and bathe Thy sullied bird of paradise in the sunrays of wisdom and the sweet-singing waters of peace.

**Come to me
in a tangible
human form**

(From a song
by Ramprasad *)

Will that day dawn for me, O
Divine Mother, when my utterance of Thy Name will bring
a flood of tears to inundate the
banks of my ignorance and end
the drought in my heart? Then in the lake of my
gathered tears will grow the luminous lotus of
wisdom, forever dispelling my darkness.

O All-Pervading Cosmic Mother, come to me
in a tangible human form! Thy face of infinite
kindness alone can banish my grief.

**Come out of
the cocoon
of delusion**

Divine Mother, ever art Thou
silently telling us: "You have
long remained in the cocoon of
wrong beliefs. Emerge before
the arrival of the silkman, Death! Cut the cords of
comfort-loving habits that hold you in a silken
prison.

"Refuse to remain a worm of error, wrapped in
thoughts of weakness. Come out of the cocoon of
delusion! By spiritual aspirations, transform your-
self into a bright moth of eternity.

"Decorate with suns and star dust your omnipresent wings of Self-realization. Glide through
the skies of infinity, attracting all beauty lovers
toward the Most Beautiful."

* See glossary.

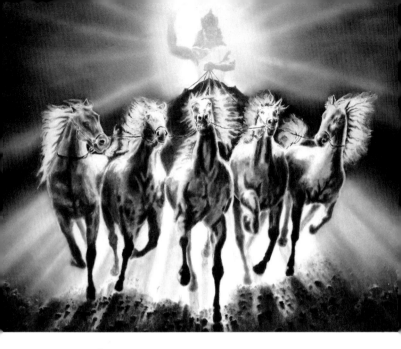

Guide me, O Soul Charioteer!
(Adapted from a passage in the Bhagavad Gita)

Teach me, O Lord, to conquer the self by the Self. May I never permit the blind ego in me to obstruct the soul.

Bless me, that I willingly appoint the soul as the body's only charioteer. May the divine driver, with its perfect discrimination, control the five fiery steeds of my senses, hold firmly the reins of my mind, and triumphantly take my little chariot on the wheels of right discipline over the speedway of incarnations.

O King of Kings, after the last lap of the final race I shall ride a chariot of Thine infinite light!

Universal daily prayer for divine guidance

O Father, Mother, Friend, Beloved God! I will reason, I will will, I will act; but lead Thou my reason, will, and activity to the right things that I should do.

Help me to win the battle of life

O Eternal Conqueror! teach me to train noble qualities within me—soldiers of calmness and self-control.

Be Thou their Divine General, like Krishna of yore, in the battle against the dark foes: anger, ingratitude, untruthfulness.

May I raise over the realm of my life Thy flag of invincible righteousness.

Overcoming my enemies: bad habits

Fierce foes, obstinate habits of restlessness, have entrenched themselves in the territory of my mind. May I overcome my enemies, bent on robbing me of my wealth of peace.

Lead Thou my battling-power to victory!

Happiness is our birthright

May we realize, O Lord, that we cannot be happy until we seek satisfaction in spiritual progress, guarding our peace of mind from all influences that would destroy it. Let us understand that happiness comes not by aimlessly thinking about it but by striving to express it in all our moods and actions.

No matter what tasks we are performing, teach us to feel the divine undercurrent, the hidden river of bliss, ever flowing beneath the sands of our myriad thoughts and the rocky soil of our difficulties.

May we be secretly joyous in spite of all adverse circumstances, knowing that happiness is our birthright, our divine "buried treasure." Guide us to find in the soul the riches beyond the dreams of kings.

May my love for Thee be unfading

O Spirit, I care not if sufferings come to me or if all things are taken from me; I pray only that my love for Thee never fade through my negligence. May the taper of devotion to Thee burn forever on the altar of my memory.

I will be Thy naughty baby, O Divine Mother!

On the playground of the earth, adorned in careless grace with mountains, plains, and seas, I have frolicked long.

O Divine Mother, each time I tired of play and loudly cried for Thee, Thou didst quiet me by dropping, through one of the open windows of my selfish desires, a glittering new toy: amusements, admirers, possessions.

This time I will be Thy naughty baby; I will sob unceasingly. Never again shall I be silenced by trinkets of transient pleasures. Thou wouldst best come soon, or with my clamor* I shall rouse all creation! Thy sleeping children will wake and join me in a chorus of wails.

O Eternal Mother, forsake the busyness of Thy universal housework! I demand attention. I want no more playthings: I want Thee!

Salutation to Spirit
(From the Bhagavad Gita)

O Spirit, I bow to Thee in front of me, behind me, on the left, and on the right. I bow to Thee above and beneath me. I bow to Thee within and without, O Lord Omnipresent!

---

* "Because of his importunity. . . He will give him." — Luke 11:8.

Keep me away from evil Bless me, that I hear no evil, see no evil, speak no evil, inhale no evil, touch no evil, feel no evil, think no evil, and dream no evil.

Lead me to the royal highway of realization Let me be Christian, Jew, Hindu, Buddhist, or Moslem; I care not what my religion or race or nationality be, so long as I win my way to Thee!

May I not wander on labyrinthine paths of religious formalities. O Lord, set Thou my feet on the one royal highway—realization of the Self; the road that leads straight to Thee.

May I exude only sweetness Teach me to be like the ripe orange which, though crushed and bitten, fails not to impart its innate sweetness.

Battered by unkindness, lashed by cruel criticism, or wounded by misunderstanding, may I unceasingly exude only the fragrance of love.

Like soap flakes which, when beaten, give out cleansing suds, may I, hard-pounded by ingratitude, offer to all the purifying foam of my deepest wisdom.

May our hearts repeat Thy Name O Utter Innocence! we are not worthy to invoke Thee. We have long indulged in worldly speech. Now with soiled lips we are calling Thee.

No matter what our activities, let us hear our soul speaking of Thee. O God, O Father! may our hearts ceaselessly repeat Thy wondrous Name.

Restore our transparency The sunbeams of Thy love shine with equal ardor on all members of Thy cosmic family —the prophet, the hero, the moth, and me.

It is man's own fault that he has become opaque through dullness. Teach us to wipe away the mists of error from our mirror of right understanding.

The arms of our spiritual resistance are weak. O Lord, switch Thy power into our limbs, that we may cleanse away the dark vapors which have settled on our transparency and prevented the free entry of Thy light. May we be bright unmarred mirrors, reflecting Thee.

O Spirit, reveal Thyself as Thou art

O Spirit, Thou art just behind my vision, with which I see Thine outward beauty. Thou art just behind my hearing, with which I listen to the medley of earth sounds. Thou art just behind my touch, with which I feel the objects of Thy world.

Thou art just behind the veil of Nature's splendors. In the sympathetic glances of flowers, in the zest of sustaining food, and in all Thine other bounties lies hidden the essence of Thy Being, Thine eternal sweetness.

As I invoke Thee, Lord, Thou art just behind my awe-trembling voice. Thou art just behind the mind with which I pray. Thou art just behind my deepest feelings. Thou art just behind my sacred thoughts. Thou art just behind my cravings for Thee. Thou art just behind my meditations. Thou art just behind my tender love.

Wilt Thou not come out from behind the screens of human feelings and creation's elaborate displays? O Inscrutable by Mortals! open my divine eye that sees Thee as Thou art.

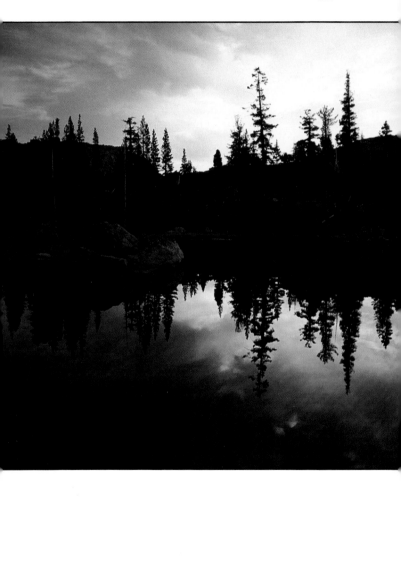

I adore Thee in the language of love

May I behold Thee, O Cosmic Mother, with my physical eyes and with the single eye* of the soul.

My wordless chants of yearning for Thee sing in cadence with my heart throbs. I bring to Thee my bouquets of devotion, activity, and knowledge; and adore Thee in the language of love: secret whispers, silent intuitive communion, and inner tears of meditative bliss.

Bless me, that my five senses encounter only goodness
(Inspired by the Hindu scriptures)

Bless me, O Lord, that I behold nothing but goodness and purity. Protect me, that I hear only inspiring speech and the beauty of devotional songs. Give me Thy grace, O Fragrant Spirit! that I inhale only odors that remind me of Thee. May I taste nothing but simple wholesome food. Let everything I touch recall to soul memory Thy sanctifying touch.

* See *spiritual eye* in glossary.

The caravan of my prayers is moving onward
The caravan of my prayers is moving toward Thee. It has been delayed now and then by blinding sandstorms of despondency.

As I lead the sacred procession I glimpse afar an oasis of Thy silent encouragement. My spirits revive; I redouble my efforts to reach Thee. May I dip my thirsty lips of faith into Thy bliss well and drink deep!

Thy simple song of joy
Volumes of Thy savior voice pour through the ether, available to human radios. Ears deafened by the static of sense pleasures cannot tune in Thy seraphic sermons.

O Blessed Broadcaster, may our mind instruments, now unreceptive to Thee, become attuned by our delicate adjustments of the dial of divine discernment.

Teach us to catch Thy highest strains: the simple song of joy.

In the garden of my life Cast unceasingly the seeds of Thy blessings into the prayer-plowed soil of my heart. May they grow into plants bearing precious fruits of Self-realization.

Let every vine of my activities wear clusters of joy. Teach me to press divine wine from the daily ripened grapes of little joys.

On each thorny bush of my trials mayest Thou grow fadeless flowers of spiritual understanding.

Thou hast many Names I say my prayers on beads of love, strung together with everlasting threads of devotion. I hold to no single Name—God, Spirit, Brahma, Allah, Heavenly Father, Divine Mother—for All are Thine.

I invoke Thee sometimes as Christ, Krishna, Shankaracharya,* Mohammed, Buddha, Moses, and other prophets; for I know Thou hast delighted, and wilt ever delight, in revealing Thyself in different forms.

In Thy cosmic play on the stage of the centuries, in Thy myriad appearances, Thou didst take many Names; but Thou hast only one Nature: Perennial Joy.

* See glossary.

Thou dost ever behold me

O Sleepless Seer of All! Thou dost behold me through the eyes of the constant sun and the moodful moon. With omnipresent gaze Thou art watching me through the myriad pores of space and through the twinkles of night-awakened stars.

With the touch of the vagrant breeze Thou dost caress me. In my loving thoughts of Thee and Thy children Thou art showering on me the silent soothing rain of Thine affection.

Prayer for supply of immediate needs

Divine Father, this is my prayer: I care not what I permanently possess, but give me power to acquire at will whatever I daily need.

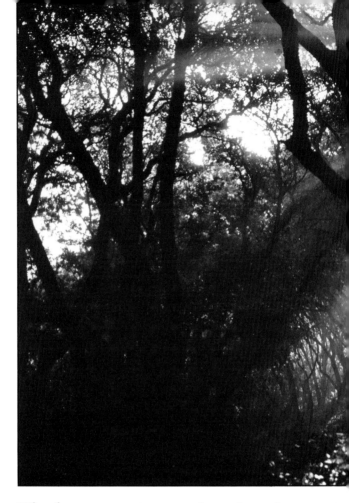

Why dost Thou seem so far away?

O Heavenly Father, Thou art just behind my prayer; why dost Thou seem so far away?

Intimations of Thy presence tremble through my feelings, and glimpses of Thee flash in my sacred thoughts; yet Thou seemest distant.

Remove the veil between us; come, Spirit, come! I yearn to know Thee and to hear Thy voice.

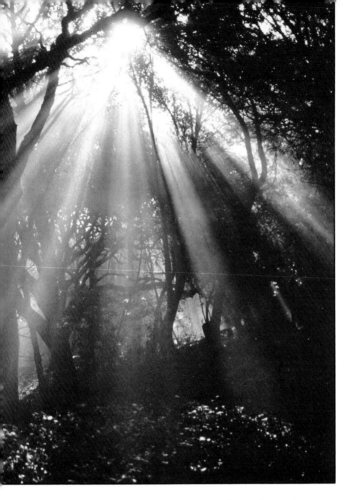

When I pray to Thee I want to realize that Thou art listening. Show me the way to reach Thee!

Darkness vanishes before Thy light O Divine Teacher, let me realize that though the gloom of my ignorance be age-old, with the dawn of Thy light the darkness will vanish as though it had never been.

Prayer for the Great Enlightenment

O August God, Beloved Father, Oversoul of the Universe, Spirit of Spirits, Friend of Friends! unravel for me the mystery of my existence. Teach me to worship Thee in breathlessness,* in sleeplessness, in deathlessness.

In the stillness of my soul, possess me; may I be conscious of Thine immortal presence in and around me. I yearn to know Thee, O Secondless, O True Unique!

Hasten Thou the day

With the dawn of Thy coming the buds of my devotion will burst into glorious bloom.

O Lord, hasten Thou the day when I may weave an amaranthine garland of those flowers and place it at Thy feet!

* See "breath" in glossary.

Prayer before taking food

Heavenly Father, receive this food; make it holy. Let no impurity of greed defile it. The food comes from Thee; it is for Thy temple. Spiritualize it. Spirit to Spirit goes.

We are the petals of Thy manifestation; but Thou art the Flower, Its life, beauty, and loveliness.

Permeate our souls with the fragrance of Thy presence.

The devotee's vow

I will conquer pride by humility, hate by love, excitement by calmness, selfishness by generosity, evil by good, ignorance by knowledge, and restlessness by the peace of meditation on Thee.

Section II

───────────

Invocations to the Manifestations of God in the Temples of Great Lives

My Guru, Sri Yukteswar

Jesus Christ

Bhagavan Krishna

Swami Shankara

Moses

Mohammed

Buddha

Mahatma Gandhi

My Guru, Sri Yukteswar   O Light of my Life! thou didst spread wisdom's glow over my soul path. Centuries of darkness vanished before the luminous shafts of thy help.

As a naughty baby* I had cried for my Mother Divine, and She came as thee — Swami Sri Yukteswar.† At that meeting, O my Guru, a sacred spark flew from thee; and the fagots of my God-cravings, gathered through incarnations, ignited and blazed into bliss. At thy flaming, golden touch all my questions were answered.

As a response to my soul cries, after years of waiting I found thee. Our hearts trembled with an omnipresent thrill. Beloved Guru,† we met in this life because we had met before.

If all the gods are wroth, and yet thou art satisfied with me, I am safe in the fortress of thy pleasure. And if all the gods protect me by the parapets of their blessings, and yet I receive not thy benediction, I am an orphan, left to pine spiritually in the ruins of thy displeasure.

O Guru, thou didst lift me out of the land of bewilderment into the paradise of peace. My slumber of sorrow is ended, and I am awake in joy.

Dissolving forever our finitude, together we shall merge in the Infinite Life.

* See page 111.   † See glossary.

O Immortal Teacher, I bow to thee as the speaking voice of silent God. I bow to thee as the divine door leading to the temple of salvation.

I lay flowers of devotion at thy feet; and before the altar of thy guru, Lahiri Mahasaya,* harbinger of modern yoga; and of his Master, deathless omnipresent Babaji.*

Come to me, O Christ, as the Good Shepherd

O Christ, beloved Son of God! thou didst embark on a storm-tossed sea of prejudiced minds. Their cruel thought waves lashed thy tender heart.

Thy trial on the Cross was an immortal victory of humility over force, of soul over flesh. May thine ineffable example hearten us to bear bravely our lesser crosses.

O Great Lover of Error-Torn Humanity! In myriad hearts an unseen monument has arisen to the mightiest miracle of love—thy words: "Forgive them, for they know not what they do."

Mayest thou remove from our eyes the cataracts of ignorance, that we see the beauty of thy message: "Love even thine enemies as thyself. Sick in mind or asleep in delusion, they are still thy brothers."

O Cosmic Christ, may we, too, conquer the

* See glossary.

Satan* of dividing selfishness that prevents the gathering in sweet accord of all men in the one fold of Spirit.

As thou art Perfection, yet wert crucified, teach us not to resent the inevitable tests of life: the daily challenge to our fortitude by adversities, our self-control by temptation, and our goodwill by misunderstanding.

Purified by contemplation on thee, innumerable devotees perfume their lives with emanations from thy flower soul. O Good Shepherd! thou leadest thy countless flock to the evergreen Pastures of Peace.

Our deepest aspiration is to see the Heavenly Father with open eyes of wisdom, as thou dost; and to know like thee that we are verily His sons. *Amen.*†

* See *maya* in glossary.
† See *Aum* in glossary.

Come to me, O Krishna, as the Divine Cowherd

O Krishna,* Lord of Hindustan, I sorrowed by the lonely Yamuna River bank, where long ago thy flute notes thrilled the air and led strayed calves to safety.

O Lotus of Love, as I mused on the sad absence of thy delusion-dispelling eyes, thine invisible Spirit took form before me — materialized as though by the irresistible force of my devotion. Thy figure of sky-blue rays seemed to walk on celestial feet along the banks of my mind, leaving there lasting impresses of Self-realization.

I am one of thy calves that, once lost, learned to follow gladly thy flower footprints in the meadows of time. Listening to thy wisdom melody, I have trod the balanced path of inner calmness and outer activity. By that road thou leadest many out of dark forests of ignorance into the land of light.

Whether going forward, sidetracked, or immobilized by disbelief, all of us are creatures of thine infinite fold. Mayest thou guide us one by one to the Elysian fields of eternal beauty.

O Divine Christ-na, thou reignest forever in each heart that hears thy heavenly flute. *Aum.**

* See glossary.

Come to me as Swami Shankara

O Shankaracharya,* dazzling star in wisdom's skies! many minds once darkened by blind belief in religious formalism have learned from thee the highest path of liberation: soul perception.

Peerless exponent of *Advaita*,† we pay homage to thee. The sheep of human weaknesses flee before the leonine roar of thy Self-realization.

Thy victory chants, *I am He*, and *Thou art That* — like Christ's affirmation, *I and my Father are one* — awaken us from the stupor of materialism.

O Swami of Swamis! thou teachest us to behold the one eternal ocean of Spirit beneath the transient, melting waves of finite forms.

Thou dost worship a God not gloom-faced and revengeful but a Bestower of boons and bliss. Thou showest us the way to garner blossoming mirth from all hearts and to fill our soul vases with bouquets of songs celestial.

* Acharya, "religious teacher," is often added to Shankara's name. The *Adi* ("first") Shankaracharya, to whom this invocation is dedicated, was born many centuries ago. He reorganized the ancient Swami Order, whose leaders successively bear the title of "Shankaracharya." See glossary.

†Literally, "nonduality," oneness. Shankara's writings are lucid expositions of the ancient Vedic teachings on *Advaita* or the essential unreality of matter, the all-inclusiveness of Spirit.

Thou dost tell us that our deathless being was churned out of His sea of light; that from His oceanic joy our many lives emerge; and that, at the subsidence of desire's storm, we shall join Him in mighty cosmic laughter.

O Majestic Monist, thy smiling life has revealed to devotees the plenitude of Spirit. We bow, we bow to thee!

Come to me as Moses   O Moses, paragon of prophets! thou dost lead weary ones from the wilderness of sorrow to the Promised Land, "flowing with milk and honey."

The lips of thy life whisper to man the fervent way to set his heart ablaze, that by its transcendent glow he glimpse the Deathless Indweller.

The Lord thy God talked with thee from the "burning bush that was not consumed"; and on holy Mount Sinai He said:

"Thou art Mine instrument; ten of My holy angels have escorted thee to earth. They shall silently blow through the trumpet of all ages the changeless melody of My Ten Commandments."

May we willingly obey the eternal edicts, O Heavenly Hebrew! and transform our lives with beauty and righteousness.

O Monotheistic Moses, teach us to worship

134

wholeheartedly the one God, the sole Ruler of heaven and earth—and no other god! Then shall it be said of us, as of thee: "The Lord spake unto Moses face to face, as a man speaketh unto his friend."*

Come to me as Mohammed

O Mohammed,† inspired Prophet of God! thy lighthouse, the *Koran*,‡ directs endangered soul ships around the lethal rocks of sin to safety in the Ultimate Harbor.

Thy soldiers sing of spiritual victory as they hasten chivalrously to rescue Dame Knowledge from the tyrant, Ignorance.

Thou warnest thy flock not to follow mirages in deserts of sense pleasures, but to browse in rich pastures of inner joy.

* Exodus 33:11.
† See glossary.
‡ The Moslem (Islamic) Bible.

Thou hast instituted the dawn-to-dusk fast during the month of Ramadan, that Spirit be attracted to the purified temple of man and offer him nectar and ambrosia.

Thy followers observe thy ban against liquors and opiates, which impair the mind and prevent divine perceptions. Thou pointest out that man's desire for intoxicants is a misguided craving for the life-transforming rejuvenator made in the *Namaz* * wine press of prayer.

With iconoclastic zeal thou dost prohibit the religious use of images and symbols; extolling, rather, simple inward worship of omnipresent Formless Spirit.

O Mohammed, to the war-drum beat of *Allah-o-Akbar* ("God is the Greatest!"), drive away from us the Satan of matter worship. With that sacred battle cry may we rout all invading thoughts of fear and limitations. *Amin*.†

* The chief prayer of the Moslems.
† See *Aum* in glossary.

Come to me as Buddha

Lord Buddha,* like a vein of shining ore in rocks of a gloomy gorge, thy message of mercy illumines a cruel world. O Heart of Pity, one day, to save a lamb from sacrifice, thou didst offer thine own body.

Loftiest Soarer in Renunciation's Skies! beneath thy God-lifted eyes the inner kingdom of ego faded away into invisibility. Thou didst forever forsake meadows of sense comforts, rivers of greed, prickly cacti of selfish worries, tall trees of temporal ambition, and gaunt deserts of desires.

Thine entire being was irrevocably set on attaining Transcendence—*Nirvana*. Under a banyan tree† thou didst make an unbreakable tryst with Spirit:

> *Beneath the banyan bough*
> *On sacred seat I take this vow:*
> *"Until life's mystery I solve*
> *Until I gain the Priceless Lore,*
> *Though bones and fleeting flesh dissolve,*
> *I'll leave this posture nevermore."*

Thy solemn thoughts still roam in the ether searching for ecstasy-tuned minds.

* See glossary.

† The pipal or *bo* tree, a variety of banyan, in Buddh Gaya, Bihar, India, under which Lord Buddha attained the Great Illumination.

Thou Symbol of Sympathy, Incarnation of Compassion! give us thy determination, that with urgency we, too, pursue Truth. Teach us to seek the Sovereign Remedy, as Thou didst, for the ills of mankind.

May thy blessings, O Buddha, help all mortals to attain the Great Awakening!

Gandhi, the Mahatma— "great soul"

O Gandhi!* the masses well named thee Mahatma, "great soul." By thy presence, many prisons became temples. Silenced, thy voice yet seemed to grow more powerful and to ring around the world. Thy message of victory through *satyagraha* ("holding to truth") touched the conscience of mankind.

Through thy reliance on God, not cannons, thou didst accomplish a feat unparalleled in history: the freeing of a vast nation from foreign rule, without hatred or bloodshed.

As thou didst sink, dying, to the ground — three bullets from a madman's gun in thy frail, fast-worn body — thy hands rose effortlessly in a sweet gesture of forgiveness. Innocent artist thou wert all the days of thy life; and, at the moment of

* See glossary.

death, thou becamest a supreme artist. All the sacrifices of thy selfless life made possible that final loving gesture.

Just as the Lord employs love, not His miraculous powers, to discipline man, so didst thou disdain the ways of force and place thy faith in the silent power of righteousness.

O Simple Saint of Truth, warriors of the future shall seriously study and finally understand thy teaching: The essential enemies of man are not his brothers—children of Spirit, the One Father; but his own ego foes, born of mortal ignorance.

Nations now distracted by political selfishness, greed, deceptions, and preparations for wars shall someday listen with open hearts to thy prophetic words:

"Nonviolence has come among men and it will live. It is the harbinger of the peace of the world."

SECTION III

———

CHILDREN'S PRAYERS

Thou art my Well-Wisher

Dear Heavenly Father, while I sleep Thou dost come to me as Peace. When I awake Thou dost come to me as Joy. When I love my friends Thou dost come to me as Love.

When I run, Thou dost run with me. When I play, Thou dost enjoy Thyself, too. When I think, Thou dost think with me. When I will, Thou dost give me the power to will.

Teach me to play rightly, to think rightly, to will rightly, and to behave rightly. I want to please Thee who art within me. I love to be guided by Thee, for Thou art my greatest Well-Wisher.

Thou art Peace and Silence

Dear Father, teach me to understand the wisdom I hear. May I enjoy my lessons at school. Help me to practice in my daily life all the good I learn.

May I feel Thee as Peace and Silence when I close my eyes. I love to pray to Thee and to talk to Thee. I know Thou art ever listening.

I bow to Thy Spirit within my heart.

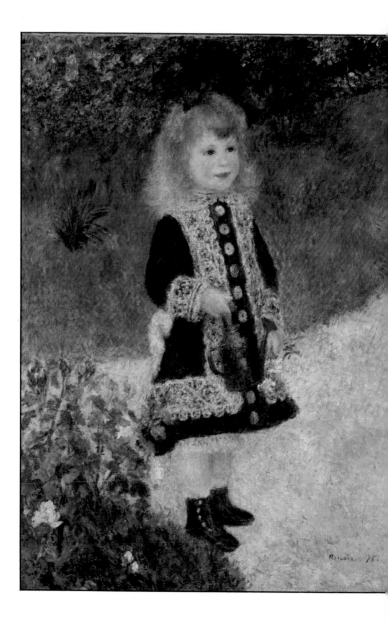

May I make others happy

Divine Mother, teach me to love others and to serve them. I want my friends to keep their promises to me, so help me always to be true to my own word.

May I make my parents happy, my teachers happy, and my playmates happy. I will find my happiness in their joy.

Thou art plainly present

Divine Father, when I dance in the waves at the seashore or in the brook, I am dancing with Thee. Every day I see Thee painting the sky in bright colors. I watch Thee clothe the bare soil with green grass. Thou art in the warmth of sunshine. Oh, Thou art so plainly present everywhere! I bow to Thee.

Giving smiles to everyone

Loving Lord, may I give cheerful smiles to all. Teach me not to laugh at others. May I not hurt anyone, in any way. Just as I myself wish to be happy, so I want to make others happy.

Thou hast no body Dear God, Thou hast no body; Thou art Spirit. By remaining formless and invisible, Thou canst be present everywhere at once.

May I watch Thee at work in the beautiful world of Nature. Let me see Thee in the clouds, in the trees, in the hills.

Thou hast made all the flowers, all the birds, all the animals, and all the people. Thou didst form the heavens and the earth. I bow to Thee.

Thou art the Cause of all Dear God, the sun comes to give us light. The moon comes in the darkness to shine on us. The seasons come to grow the crops so all Thy children may have food. Thou art the Cause of all this goodness. I bow to Thee.

Thou art Love Dear Heavenly Father, my parents love me because Thou dost love me. My relatives and friends love me because Thou dost love me.

I love my country and all other lands because Thou hast made them. Thou didst create the whole world out of Thy love. I bow to Thee.

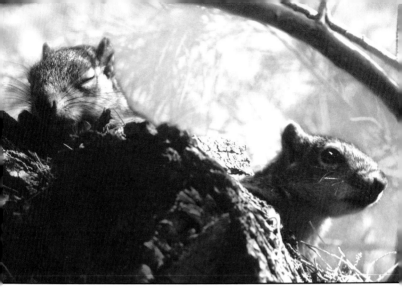

**May I find
Thy love
in all**

Divine Mother, teach me to love all my little friends. By loving them, may I find Thy love in everyone I meet.

I want to love those who love me. I want to offer my love to those who do not seem to love me. I enjoy loving all, for they are my brothers and sisters.

**Thou art my
Best Friend**

Dear God, I know Thou art Love, because my mother and my father love me. Thou art my Heavenly Father and my Heavenly Mother.

My friends love me, for Thou art present in their hearts. Thou art my Best Friend. Thou art my Divine Teacher. Even as Thou lovest me, teach me to love Thee.

I bow to Thee everywhere

Loving Lord, I thank Thee for Thy wonderful water. When I am thirsty I drink it because Thou hast made it, clear and cool, for me. When I am soiled by play, I bathe in Thy water and feel refreshed.

When the sunshine falls on my face, I thank Thee for Thy warm loving touch. When the clouds cover the sky, and then the sun comes out from behind the clouds, I know Thou art playing hide-and-seek with me.

I bow to Thee in the water, in the sunshine, and in all other daily joys. I bow to Thee at dawn, at noontime, in the afternoon, and in the quiet evening.

My Home is Heaven

Dear Father, I came from Thy Home in Heaven, to play a while on earth. Someday I shall return to my Real Home with Thee.

I want Thee to welcome me with open arms, so in the world I will keep myself clean and holy. To do this I will constantly think of Thee. I bow at Thy feet. *Aum, Amen*.

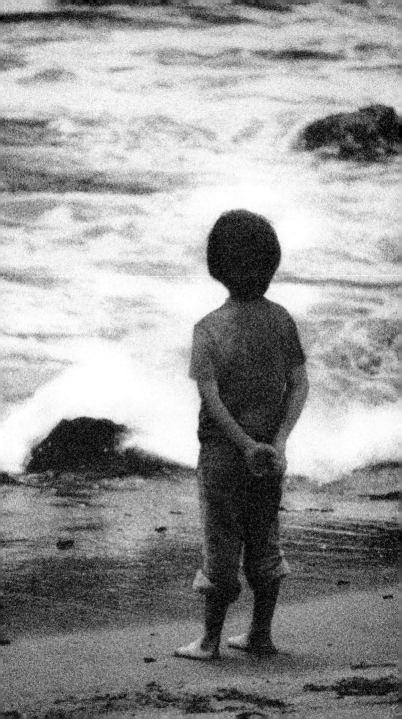

SECTION IV

EXPERIENCES IN
SUPERCONSCIOUSNESS
AND
MESSAGES TO DEVOTEES

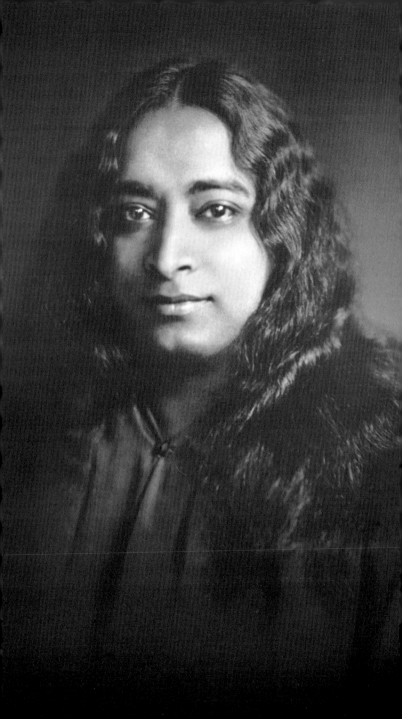

Whispers from Eternity   The Eternal Voice softly said to me: "Through thy slumber of ages I whispered, 'Wake thyself!' Thou hast forsaken thy sleep, so now I say, 'Wake thy brothers!' Work thou with Me, that all men hear My word."

"I shall broadcast Thy message," I promised. "And when I leave my earthly form, I shall borrow Thine omnipresent voice to murmur within each receptive heart: 'Oh, listen to His soul-solacing songs!'"

My countless brothers! I shall wait for all. As they slowly travel in a seemingly endless procession toward the blissful goal of Self-realization, through *Whispers from Eternity* I shall gently say: "Awake! Following His ever calling voice, let us go Home together."

O Fairy Song of Love Everlasting

I tune the harpstrings of my heart to play an old song newly — the story of my first-born love.

O Spirit, I would offer Thee fresh notes from the virginal soul; original variations on the change-less theme of my adoration.

My hymn waves dance to the cosmic rhythms of Thine Ocean and float me on billows of bliss to Thy terminal shores.

O Lullaby of the Sea Serene! ever croon to me thy devotion chant to the Divine Eternal Mother.

O Fairy Song of Love Everlasting! rock me in thy cradle of melody and bring me sleep on Her bosom of peace.

"Be happy, My child!"

In a time of misfortune I heard Thy voice, saying:[*] "The sun of My protection shines equally on thy brightest and thy blackest hours.

"Have faith and smile! *Sadness is an offense against the blissful nature of Spirit.* Let My life-transforming light appear through the transparency of smiles. By being happy, My child, thou dost please Me."

[*] In my native language, Bengali.

Welcome, O Majestic Personage! From the vault of memory I removed the sacred treasure of bonds and promissory notes given to me by Thee. I cashed them into love's gold and built on spacious grounds of my soul a palace worthy of Thy throne of bliss. Now I await Thy coming.

O Majestic Personage, Thou art approaching my joy-bedecked heart! Diamond chips of my broken dreams, long darkness hidden, glitter in the flash of Thy visit. From my rapt being, silent chants of praise flow insuppressibly.

Accept Thou the welcoming garlands I have fashioned from undying flowers of my devotion.

Thou art the Fountain of Love Thou art the Fountain of Love, heavenly and earthly. Thou art the protecting father; Thou art the mother, showering infinite kindnesses. Thou art the little child, lisping love to his parents. Thou dost manifest Thyself in the wholehearted surrender of one lover to the other. Thou dost purify the servant by respect for his master; Thou dost cement the fondness of friends.

Thou hast bathed me in the spray of all loves. With the full gamut of feeling, with the subtleties and delicate distinctions of the various types of affection I have come to love Thee, O God Adorable!

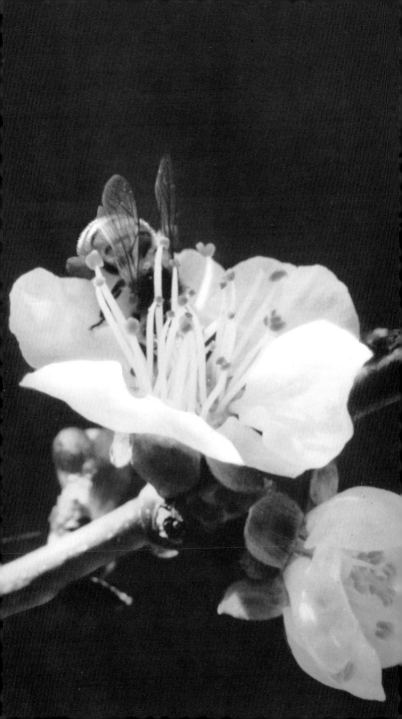

The blue-rayed lotus of Thy feet   O Divine Mother, the bee of my mind is engrossed in the blue-rayed lotus of Thy feet. I drink the nectar of Thy tender love. This royal bee of Thine sips only from the blossom that exudes Thy perfume.

Denying myself the honey of sense pleasures, flying far above ephemeral gardens of idle fancy, at last I have found Thine ambrosial lotus of light.

I was Thy busy bee, wandering in the fields of incarnations, attracted by odors from flowers of countless experiences. I roam no more, for Thy fragrance has quenched the perfume thirst of my soul.

Memories   Thou hast given me recollection of past incarnations in which I loved and sought Thee. Whether on earth or in the astral world I pursued Thee. Dost remember when I met Thee in the bower of the Milky Way? and worshiped Thee in the beauty of protean forms of creation?

I am Thy little bee that yearned for the nectar of happiness. Greedily I drank from many blossoms of transient love and capricious Nature. But when I came upon the eternal sweetness of Thy lotus heart, I hummed with desires no more.

O Wine of Centuries!

I attuned myself to Thee, and now my life is an unbroken inspiration. Thy bliss inundates me in my wakeful state, slumber, dreamless sleep, and deep *turiya.* *

Vision after sublime vision! Oh, what has become of me? Indescribable divine intoxications wavelike overwhelm me.

O Consecrated Wine of Uncounted Centuries, I have found Thee—I have found Thee at last! Give me Eternity to taste all Thy sweetness.

---

* Literally, in Sanskrit, the "fourth" or superconscious state. Human beings experience three states: waking, dream-broken slumber, and dreamless sleep. The latter, even when brief, is revivifying; man is then unconsciously resting in his soul nature.

Few persons explore the fourth or unrestricted region of mind. Persistent yogis and all other great devotees of God enter the *turiya* state: conscious, unforgettable realizations of Spirit.

Thou didst Parental blood in my veins and
baptize me milk of mother breasts were the
in the flood waters that baptized me in the
of Thy grace consciousness of flesh.

My soul, confined in a fragile frame, cried for release. Within the fenced garden of the charming senses no more I loved to abide.

Then the cloud of Thy silence burst, O Lord! Its merciful drops rained upon me and became a flood of Thy grace. The river of Thy Spirit overran the boundaries of my soul and baptized me in blissful waters of eternity. The little bubble of my being dissolved and melted in Thine omnipresent sea.

The seraphic The magic wand of meditation
strains touches all sounds, melting
of *Aum* them into the primal *Aum*.*
It courses through the stars, through the earth, through the waters. O Spirit, reveal Thyself to me as *Aum, Aum,* the call to prayer of the cosmos.

All tissues of my body, all filaments of my nerves now sing seraphic strains of *Aum*!

* See glossary.

Doors everywhere   O Father, when I was blind I found not a door that led to Thee. Thou hast healed my eyes; now I discover doors everywhere: the hearts of flowers, the voices of friendship, memories of lovely experiences.

Each gust of my prayer opens a new entrance to the vast temple of Thy presence.

I beheld Thee hiding in a flower   I looked at a flower and prayed. Suddenly, O Spirit, I beheld Thee hiding there. It exhaled the perfume of Thy presence. The blush of Thine innocence colored its petals; the gold of Thy wisdom shone in its heart.

The slender stem and delicate green calyx were upheld by Thine omnipresent power. The mystery of life and immortality lay in the pollen; and Thine infinite touch transfigured the breast of the bee tasting Thy sweetness.

Oh, reveal to me the wonders of creation, Thine endless secrets that even the tiniest roadside weed bears in its bosom!

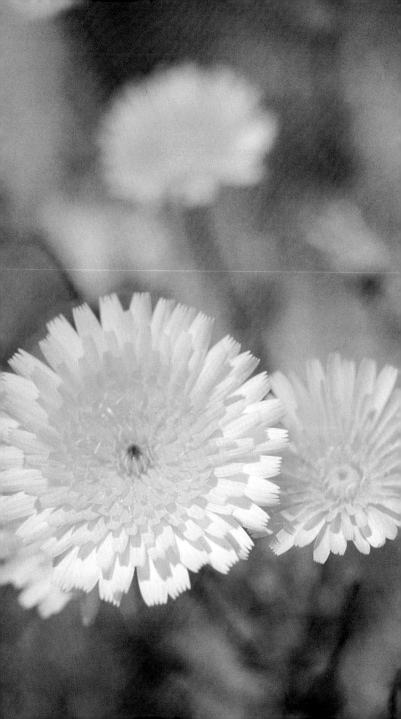

A prayer of loyalty [*] In sickness or health, in sorrow or joy, in poverty or prosperity, in disaster or security, in death or life, I stand unalterably, immutably, unchangeably loyal, devoted, and loving to Thee, my Heavenly Father! forever, forever, and forever.

Thy light in the sunless ocean depths My mind submarine submerged beneath the surface waves of earthly ambitions. With miraculous, meditation-acquired powers it dived to the abyssal waters of the inner ocean.

Moving whalelike, my faith-guided mind submarine searched for Thee through sunless canyons and stark mountain gorges. It looked for Thee in silence regions, unexplored by mortals: the final chasms and nethermost hollows in the sea of consciousness.

Thou didst suddenly appear, O Omnipresence, revealing Thine eternal light within the age-old darkness of the deeps.

[*] Written after I had undergone at God's hands a great test.

I wear my scars as roses of courage

I have bled for Thy Name; and for Thy Name's sake I am willing ever to bleed. Like a mighty warrior, with gory limbs, injured body, wounded honor, and a thorn crown of derision, undismayed I fight on. My scars I wear as roses of courage, of inspiration to persevere in the battle against evil.

I may continue to suffer blows on my arms outstretched to help others, and receive persecution instead of love. But my soul shall ever bask in the sunshine of Thy blessings, O Lord! Thou dost guide Thy soldier's campaigns that conquer for Thee the lands of human hearts now oppressed by sadness.

With the transfiguring sword of wisdom I smite the error foe. My army of freedom thoughts is disciplined by the divine martinet, Singlehearted Devotion to Thee. Blowing trumpets of Thy liberating Name, the battalions march into enemy-occupied territory: *maya*-deluded minds.

May the legions of light banish the despot, Darkness — usurper in man's kingdom of consciousness.

Oh, in my invasions of the continents of ignorance Thou hast ever been Commander in Chief!

In the bursts of blue brine

(Written at the seashore in Encinitas)

Picturesque beach by the Pacific, heaven of health next to Paradise! Absent, from these calm shores, the enervating vapors of lowlands and the dryness of proud hills.

In the bursts of blue brine my spirit bounds in joy. The salty spray seems to enter my bloodstream, filling to overflowing my reservoir of strength. What vital volumes of life force come to me with the ocean breeze!

Lord, as on the far horizon Thou hast knit together the fabrics of sky and sea, so mayest Thou weave infinite thoughts into the restless mind of man, that he realize his immortal immensity.

I remember, I remember!

I remember past lives in which I sought Thee — the many nights adorned with starry twinkles; the many dawns of dewy innocence; the many twilights that came in cadence with cowbells; the many years bedecked in spring blossoms, in summer zephyrs, in transparent robes of rain, and in winter's diamond icicles.

Blushing with joyous expectancy, many times have I awaited Thee!

Removing the cork of ignorance No longer is my consciousness limited to a phial of flesh, corked with ignorance. No more do I move through Thine Ocean of Spirit day and night, years, incarnations — so close, yet without contacting the Sea. No longer do I thoughtlessly dwell in Thee, knowing and feeling Thee not.

As I listened in awe to the ever expanding cosmic sound, the surging of Thy holy Name,* the vibrations removed the tight cork of delusion that had long prevented the mingling of my waters and Thine.

Now my being is consciously merged in Thine omnipresence. Having released the "I-ness" in me, I know that Thou art I; and that Thou art the souls of all.

At play with Thee In innumerable lives I have played with Thee; I have sung countless songs.

I remember Thy warm embrace whenever, after centuries, I returned home to Thee with the chill of separation on me. Again, in the present day of Thine eternity, I play with Thee and I sing Thy songs.

* See *Aum* in glossary.

164

I shall be a messenger of joy

I desire no monuments in the halls of fame. After death I shall enter countless caves of soul love and secretly inspire my brothers with dulcet spiritual thoughts.

Unknown, I shall be a gentle ghostly messenger of joy. I shall visit the dark mounds in human minds — the graves of bright aspirations. There I shall light hope candles fashioned in my nook of silence.

I play hide-and-seek with Thee

O Lord of Lila!* in the borderland between wakefulness and sleep Thou dost come to play with me, Thy servant. Floating on the ocean of Thy love for me, I dance over cosmic waves of gaiety. With laughter I play hide-and-seek with Thee.

Thy humble greatness makes me, Thine infinitesimal creature, sit on Thy vast eternal throne.

* In the Hindu scriptures creation is said to be God's playground — scene of His *lila* or loving sport with His creatures.

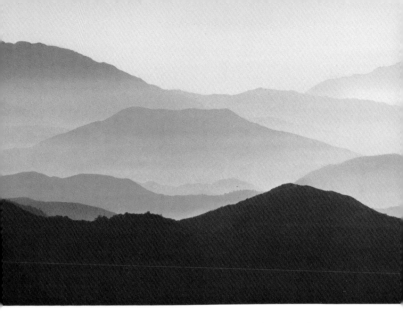

**Dreaming,
I thought
I was awake**

As we rest, and wake a little, to slumber again, so from beneath the coverlet of fleeting dreams of experiences we rise for a while and then fall asleep, to dream again of yet another chapter of earthly struggle.

On the sleigh of incarnations we slide from dream to dream. Dreaming, in a chariot of astral light we roll from life to life. Dreaming, in a vibrant physical vessel tossed by alternating waves of birth and death, we sail uncharted seas. Becalmed waters of indifference, whirlpools of activity, eddies of laughter, inexorable swells of mighty outer events—dreams all!

It was only in Thee I awoke! Then I realized that, thinking I was awake, I had been only dreaming.

O Colossal Denizen of the Deeps! I sought to catch Thee in the secret waters of supercon- sciousness. To lure Thee I used the bait of love. Its fragrance at- tracted many rare fish of sacred inspirations; the float-quill of my yearning bobbed often. But, Elu- sive Lord, every time I reeled in my line I found I had missed Thee.

With ever attentive zeal I watched. Suddenly the quill sank in fulfillment beneath the swell of Thy bliss waves.

I pulled steadily at the line; and Thou, O Co- lossal Denizen of the Deeps! didst leap into the boat of my life.

I asked Thee:
"What is sin?"
O Transcendent Teacher, in the chamber of soul stillness I asked Thee: *What is sin?*

Thine essential silence became secret articulations of my intuition; I understood Thine answer:

Sin is the rebel king, Ignorance.

The originator and pioneer of all suffering, Ignorance is the mysterious root of the tree of ill-health, the source of every type of mental inefficiency, and the primal cause of man's soul blindness.

Stealthily reigning within unenlightened minds, the evil Emperor maintains sinister courtiers: inertia, greed, false convictions, selfish ambitions, ignoble thoughts.

They destroy all crops of nourishing spirituality. In many men the harvest of faith, ripe for the reaping, has been cruelly trampled down by the dragoons of doubt.

May we dethrone Darkness by witnessing within us Thy triumphal coronation, O Eternal Sovereign of Light!

The immortalizing rays of Spirit

Entering the infinite temple of silence, I switched off the dazzling diverting lights in the sense bulbs: sight, hearing, taste, smell, and touch.

I commanded the noisy body cleaner of breath to cease; I bade my heart not to enslave my cells with the physical food of blood; for within me Thy footstep resounded, O Cosmic Mother, as Thou camest with a chalice of divine rays.*

Oh, feed me forever with Spirit Sustenance! The brain, the heart, the cells will no longer decay but with transcendent life be immortalized.†

---

* The first two paragraphs describe the effect of a yogic technique, taught in the *Self-Realization Fellowship Lessons,* that disconnects the sense telephones from outside stimuli, quiets the breath and heartbeat, and stills the thoughts. Only thus, in a temple of silence, may man approach his Maker. "Be still, and know that I am God."— Psalms 46.10.

† This is a prophetic passage. The Mortuary Director of Forest Lawn Memorial-Park, Glendale, testified that after Paramahansa Yogananda's death his flesh "manifested a phenomenal state of immutability .... No odor of decay emanated from his body at any time." See page 201. *(Publisher's Note)*

Thy *danse macabre*   Thou lovest the wild dance of destruction,* O Cosmic Mother! Thou dost shatter frail mortal frames to show us, smilingly, that our souls are immortal, invulnerable.

In Thy relentless, mercy-inspired *danse macabre* Thou dost fling away our outworn bodily garments and shake loose the long-encrusted mud of our delusions.

Because Thou art pleased by the crematory rites of dissolution, I have burnt in Thy furnace of wisdom all my desires and weaknesses. Nothing of my finiteness remains; Thou hast annihilated the last vestige.

O Whimsical Woman, Divine Mistress of Contrasting Moods! now Thou dost dance with me Thy harmonious rhythms of creation and preservation.

Let all rest in the shade of my peace   The breeze of Thy love wafts through me, O Father! The leaves of my tree of life gently tremble in response to Thy coming. Their blissful murmur floats through the ether and calls weary ones to rest in the shade of my peace.

* See page 178.

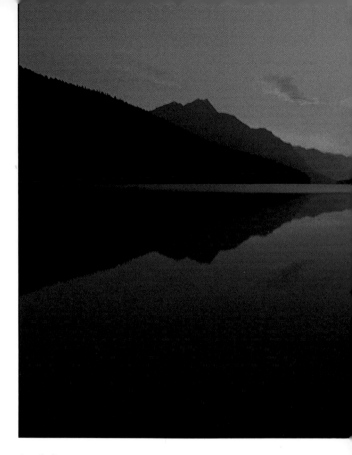

**A vision
of Christ
and Krishna**

I beheld a great blue valley encircled by mountains that shimmered jewel-like. Around opalescent peaks vagrant mists sparkled. A river of silence flowed by, diamond-bright.

And there I saw, coming out of the depths of the mountains, Jesus and Krishna walking hand in hand—the Christ who prayed by the river Jordan and the Christ-na who played a flute by the river Yamuna.

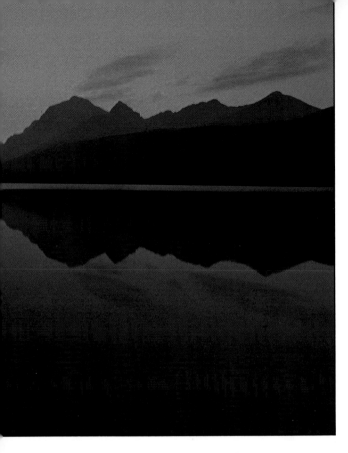

They baptized me in the radiant waters; my soul melted in fathomless depths.

Everything began to emit astral flames. My body and the forms of Christ and Krishna, the iridescent hills, the glowing stream, and the far empyrean became dancing lights, while atoms of fire flew. Finally nothing remained but mellow luminosity, in which all creation trembled.

O Spirit! in my heart I bowed again and again to Thee — Eternal Light in whom all forms commingle.

Terrors of mun-dane delusion are but dreams Wrapped in the blanket of earthly hopes, I slept long. I dreamt that I was sitting on a throne; my face wore a bouquet of smiles. It soon withered; one by one the petals of merriment dropped.

Then I beheld myself in rags, lying on the jagged stones of poverty. In the unrelenting grip of adversities I sobbed bitterly. My tears fell unheeded; the world passed me by in mocking silence.

My heart wailed for Thy help. Moved by the spiritual force of my unceasing pleas, Thou didst waken me at last. In joy I found myself secure in Thee, beyond the reach of bewildering dualities.

Mayest Thou awaken all other men from the world dream of smiling opulence and crying poverty. Deliver them, O Maker of Dreams! from ugly nightmares of death. Revive in them the consciousness of immortality. Bless them, that by unbroken calmness they realize the terrors of mundane delusion are but dreams.

A nightingale
of heaven
A nightingale of heaven, I have perched in the trees of many incarnations.

In the garden of the centuries I pour forth my orisons, rousing sleeping ones to awake in Thee.

I travel from one heart bower to another, giving concerts of Thy blissful songs.

I shall come to earth again and again. I yearn to attract straying birds, to teach them Thy sacred melodies, and to fly with them to Thy skies of eternal freedom.

I shall
swim in the
sea of souls
At one with Thee, O Spirit, I shall be the universal throb of life. I shall swim in the sea of souls. Dancing on the waves of mankind's sacred feelings, I shall besprinkle all with divine delight. From the Himalayas of Heaven I shall start a world avalanche of noble desires.

I shall be all teardrops shed in sympathy for others. I shall be present in the golden silence of saints and in the budding hopes of rosy minds.

O Faithful Fulfiller of Wishes! when my immortal spark commingles with Thine Infinite Light I shall twinkle through all eyes.

The honeycomb of my heart

In the summer days of life I gather nectar from blossoms of sweet qualities that grow in the garden of human souls.

I store the essence of tall flowers of forgiveness, of faint-scented buds of humility, and of rare blooms of lotus thoughts.

When snowflakes of wintry experiences and earthly separations swirl around me, I seek warmth and joy in the honeycomb of my heart. There I have often discovered Thee, O Bee Divine, sipping the hoarded sweetness of my devotion. In the hive hallowed by Thee I find my nook of solace.

I shall spread Thy holy Name

O Lord of Good Tidings, to broadcast Thine urgent message I shall fly from peak to cosmic peak.

Whirling in the starry dance, I shall emblazon Thy glory.

With the nebulae, over the immensities I shall spread Thy holy Name.

Timing my song with Thine, I shall chant in the humming atoms.

I shall penetrate human hearts with darts of Thy love, and silence the songbirds with the wondrous story of Thy Being.

Invincible Lion of the Self   A cub of the Divine Lion, somehow I found myself confined in a sheepfold of frailties and limitations. Fear-filled, living long with sheep, day after day I bleated. I forgot my affrighting bellow that banishes all enemy sorrows.

O Invincible Lion of the Self! Thou didst drag me to the water hole of meditation, saying: "Thou art a lion, not a sheep! Open thine eyes, and roar!"

After Thy hard shakings of spiritual urge, I gazed into the crystal pool of peace. Lo, I saw my face like unto Thine!

I know now that I am a lion of cosmic power. Bleating no more, I shake the error forest with reverberations of Thine almighty voice. In divine freedom I bound through the jungle of earthly delusions, devouring the little creatures of vexing worries and timidities, and the wild hyenas of disbelief.

O Lion of Liberation, ever send through me Thy roar of all-conquering courage!

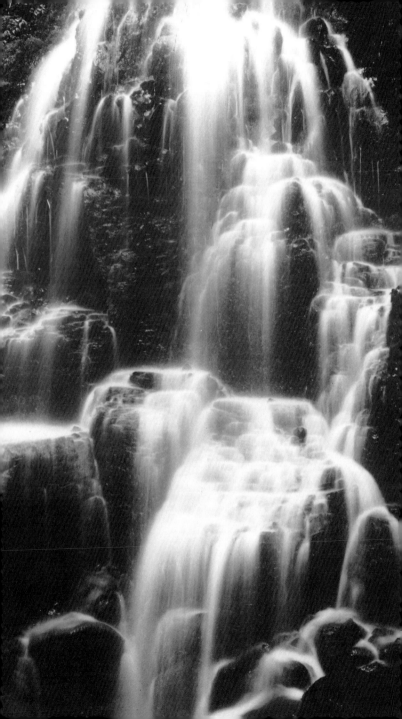

My journey's end Stumbling along the winding ways of misgivings, crossing chimerical chasms of age-old separations, racing over countless tracts of lives, dogging the steps of many ambitions, freeing myself from whirlpools of sadness and pleasure, at last I am at my journey's end.

I look upon my bygone travail with joy; from every rock of past agony now flows a spring of blissful tears. In the sacred waters of those tears of love for Thee, daily I baptize myself.

At Thy touch, dumb matter speaks Because Thou camest to me, O Lord, many doors miraculously open before me. At Thy footfall, everything shines with life. Spirit-resurrected by Thy touch, dumb matter speaks. A marble floor on which I stood one day thrilled me because of Thy presence within it.

I have discovered Thy silent sanctuary, O Divine Indweller! long hidden behind a rocky fortress of seeming inaccessibility.

Incense breezes bear to me Thy perfume of bliss. On an altar stone of sacredness plays Thy fountain of joy. With palm cups uplifted in craving, I catch and drink Thy solacing waters; and realize I need thirst no more.

I beheld Thee in Thy dances of creation, preservation, and destruction

O Kali,* I bow to Thee — all-sheltering Mother Nature, ruler of time, space, form, and relativity. Invisible Spirit took shape in Thee, a visible Woman Divine.

The beauty spot of the moon is set between Thy spacious eyebrows. Clouds of eternity hide Thy face. Gusts of prophet lives blow aside momentarily Thy mystery veil, revealing to mankind glimpses of Thine ineffable beauty.

The countless worlds delineate Thy form — million-eyed, moon-garlanded, infinite in adornments and glories. In Thy changing robes are woven the dreams of creation, preservation, and destruction. On the endless etheric curtain of Thy mind a myriad cosmic dramas play. Thou dost entertain Thy good children and frighten Thy naughty ones.

O Kali Primordial, from Thy hand of creative power issue the vibrations of *Aum*, materializing in an inexhaustible, bewildering, and wondrous

---

* Kali is literally "The Dark One," and is also the feminine form of the Sanskrit word *kala*, "time" — the finite world of transitoriness. Kali is *shakti*, divine power, the kinetic aspect of Cosmic Consciousness that makes possible the endless universal unfoldments. Kali is thus the Divine Mother, the life-infusing Spirit of Nature, the "female" or fertile aspect of the Uncreated Absolute.

variety of finite forms. Another hand holds the astral sword of preservation, keeping guard over planetary rhythms and balances. Thy third hand clutches the severed head of Cosmos, symbolizing annihilation in Brahma's Night.* Thy fourth hand† stills the storm of delusion and bestows on devotees Thy rays of salvation.

Thou dost project the fabulous dream fiestas of the centuries: the pageant of human life and death, the birth and passing of civilizations, and the evolution and dissolution of solar systems.

On earth Thou art equally present in the slums of misery, the halls of festive prosperity, and the quiet shrines of wisdom.

O Pristine Mother, in the cyclic dawn of creation I beheld‡ Thee crowned with wild Nature,

---

* The Hindu scriptures conceive of creation as an eternal concept in the Divine Mind and therefore endlessly recurrent. A cycle of manifested creation (Brahma's Day) is followed, after a vast period of time, by destruction and a cycle of unmanifestation (Brahma's Night). Then another Cosmic Day dawns, followed by another Cosmic Night; and so on. See *Yuga* in glossary.

† The four hands of Kali symbolize the four rays of *Aum,* distinctive vibratory types of cosmic activity.

See *Kali* and *Aum* in glossary.

‡ These passages describe a vision in *samadhi* in which I was permitted by the Great Mother to observe Her at Her universal work.

wearing the scant garment of primitive cultures and roaming amidst unpolished minds.

In the noonday of creation I saw Thee in full activity. Thy vast body perspired as Thou, unseen, didst accomplish the tasks set by the restless ambition of Thy children. They felt the strain of struggle; scorched by their own ego blaze, men implored Thee to send cooling breezes of soul peace.

The night of total destruction approached; I beheld Thee covered ominously with mourning veils. Thou didst plunge the universe into a terrible but purifying ordeal by fire. The sun burst, belching smoke and flames; doomful quakes sundered the sky and conflagrated the stars. The worlds vanished; within Thy crucible, matter became pure, luminous.

The phenomenal spheres, that came from light,* slept as astral embers. Then, stirred by Thee, O Perennial Mother, the universe reawoke in its vibratory body of subtle flames.

The Unmanifested Infinite is hidden beneath the magic shroud of *Maya*, whilst Thou, O Exuberant Goddess of Forms, dost whirl in fantastic dances of finitude. Thy wild steps cease only when

---

* "Let there be light: and there was light."—Genesis 1:3.

Thy feet touch the transcendent breast of Thy consort, Shiva, in whom all creation has rest.*

Everywhere, O Kali, I hear Thy voice, resounding in the thunder or singing softly in the flux of atoms. I hear Thee in the symphony of spinning stars. I hear Thee, too, in the tinkling bells of little, laughing, harmonious lives. Thou art nearer to me than the throbs of my heart; and I perceive Thee on the farthest horizon of consciousness.

O Dancer of Unsearchable Caprice! Thine entrancing footsteps ever echo in my soul.

* Shiva or the Infinite is transcendent (inactive in the phenomenal worlds). He has relegated to His "consort" Kali all powers of creation, preservation, and destruction.

In ancient Hindu texts, the universe is said to vanish "when Kali's flying feet touch the breast of Shiva"; that is, when the Finite meets the Infinite. The world of appearances dissolves in Reality.

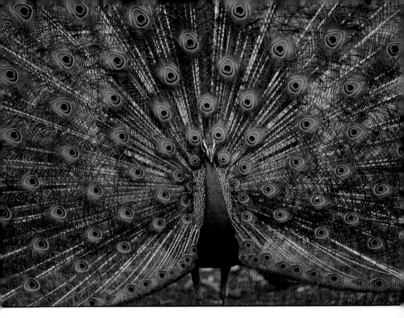

**The beauty
of Thy plan**
The drought of ignorance was
banished by the shower of Thy
blessings. The petals of the flow-
er of past-present-future opened and revealed to me
the intricate beauty of Thy plan in creation.

**Awake and
ready**
O Eternal Father, Thou hast
awakened me; can I ever fall
again into slumber? Yet if sleep
should steal over me, promise that Thou wilt
rouse me!

The terrors of the dreamland of life are forgotten now. My sorrow Thou hast changed into
tears of joy. My joys are blazing into bliss. My body
temple is filled with light. Thy rays prevent my
wisdom eyes from drooping. I thank Thee, O Lord,
for keeping me always awake and ready!

A butterfly of eternity

With the sharpness of my will I tore to shreds the stifling chrysalis of ignorance.

Now I am a butterfly of eternity, gracefully sweeping through the empyrean. Bespangled with whirling galaxies, in joy I spread my Nature wings. Behold my deathless beauty!

Cut the dark threads of thy shrouding fears, O my brothers! Follow me in the flight to Him.

Thou hast satisfied my soul hunger

O All-Pervading Spirit, the breeze of Thine inspiration has banished all clouds; the firmament of my mind is clear. With purified eyes I behold everywhere only Thee.

The sunshine of Thy joy penetrates to the innermost depths of my being. With the hunger of ages I feed upon Thy light.

By Thy grace and by my constant wakefulness, may this bliss be mine forever and forever.

The lark that drinks Thy raindrops

I am Thy lark that ascended the skies of Thy cosmic presence, ever seeking the raindrops of truth. Deeply I prayed that Thou release from cruel clouds of silence Thy mercy showers. Parched and craving, gratefully I drank each sacred drop of perceptions of Thee.

I yearned to feel Thee within and without. My age-old thirst ceased only when Thy touch cooled my fiery soul and zeal-warmed body.

The drought of despondency has passed. The dryness of my unfulfillment was banished by Thy downpour of peace. Now I soar serenely, cascading Thy song of contentment.

I am Thy lark, imbibing only the secret waters of solace that fall unfailingly from the heavens of Thy Being.

What bliss at the sight of Thy light!

As I muse on Thee a thrilling fountain spray lightninglike spreads from my heart to all cells of my body, saturating them with divine devotion. I seek to enter the inmost heaven of Thy presence.

The soul's secret door suddenly opens; and, oh, what bliss I feel at the sight of Thy light!

The forest of delusion ablaze

Unhappy in the forest of delusion, I kindled fagots of self-discipline; but the fire only smoldered.

Urgently I prayed. Thou didst come and set ablaze a few of my frailties. The flames quickly spread in the bushes of error, entered the thick underbrush of prickly desires, and reached the tall trees of vanities. The vast jungle of my ignorance was consumed in the fires of Thy light.

I thank Thee, O Divine Incendiary! May all Thine other children learn to call upon Thee for instant help.

Thy station, JOY From Thy station, JOY, I hear daily Thine ineffable shrill-soft* tones, dear and familiar.

At first I tried to tune Thee in from so far, far away; Thy program seemed beyond the reception of the tiny instrument of my mind. But after I had made many fine touches on the dial of meditation, Thou didst come in on sudden etheric wings.

Thou wert singing a melody of earth's goodness and the nobility in all hearts.

Thy pristine song gushed through me To hear Thee, O Guardian Angel of All, with soft touches of love I tuned my intuition radio.

Often in meditation I listened to the dulcet melodies of Those close to Thee, to majestic soul symphonies, to full strains from the vestal choir of my heart's sacred feelings, and to plaintive chants of my age-old craving for Thee.

Patiently I kept tuning my deepest percep-

* One of the characteristic sounds of *Aum*—God in His aspect of the Holy Ghost.

tions. Then, as I nodded and almost slept, Thy pristine song gushed through me!

Now I broadcast ecstatic echoes of Thy melody of mirth. * My voice shall forever swell the chorus of Thy devotees.

---

* Man is both a receiving and a transmitting station, Paramahansa Yogananda wrote in *Autobiography of a Yogi*:

"Thoughts are no more than very subtle vibrations moving in the ether....All thoughts vibrate eternally in the cosmos. By deep concentration a master is able to detect the thoughts of any man, living or dead. Thoughts are universally and not individually rooted; a truth cannot be created, but only perceived. Any erroneous thought of man is a result of an imperfection, large or small, in his discernment....

"The human mind, freed from the disturbances or 'static' of restlessness, is empowered to perform all the functions of complicated radio mechanisms—sending as well as receiving thoughts, and tuning out undesirable ones. As the power of a radio-broadcasting station is regulated by the amount of electrical current it can utilize, so the effectiveness of a human radio depends on the degree of will power possessed by each individual....

"The will, projected from the point between the eyebrows, is the broadcasting apparatus of thought. Man's feeling, or emotional power, calmly concentrated on the heart, causes it to act as a mental radio that receives the messages of others from far and near." *(Publisher's Note)*

The wondrous eyes of Christ

One night while I was engaged in silent prayer, my sitting room in the hermitage in Encinitas became filled with an opal blue light. I beheld the radiant form of the blessed Lord Jesus.

A young man, he seemed, of about twenty-five, with a sparse beard and moustache; his long black hair, parted in the middle, was haloed by a shimmering gold.

His eyes were eternally wondrous; as I gazed, they were infinitely changing. With each divine transition in their expression I intuitively understood the wisdom conveyed. In his glorious gaze I felt the power that upholds the myriad worlds.

A Holy Grail appeared at his mouth; it came down to my lips and then returned to Jesus. After a few moments he uttered beautiful words, so personal in their nature that I keep them in my heart.

Thine approaching feet

In deep meditation I hear the blissful sound of Thine approaching feet. Their soft tread banishes from my mind all memories of earth's noisy pleasures. My finiteness slumbers, cradled in the arms of my deep perceptions of Thee.

I swept Thy wisdom's ocean for treasure

A long time ago I had a secret flashlight. A-tiptoe in the silent inner darkness, I would send a swift beam all around. Often I beheld little fish of creative ideas, entrapped by the sudden radiance.

I used them as bait to catch bigger denizens of my consciousness. But, beyond the small circle of brightness, many a good one slipped away.

From Thy perfect devotees—rich in silvery songs and gold-spun dreams—with coins of love I bought effulgent nets of soul perceptions. I joined them into a huge dragnet of woven light and swept Thy wisdom's ocean.

I hauled up spawn of goodness, minnow schools of happy feelings, long-lost treasures of divine memories—and Thyself!

Adoring Thee through all the aeons In the temple of meditation I light twin lamps of dawn and my own wakefulness. Gorgeous garlands of my devotion encircle Thy feet of omnipresence.

Thy fragrance exuding from love flowers in the vase of my heart permeates every nook of my being.

All shadows and fears of my imagination vanished at Thy light-coming, O Lord! Thou hast roused me forever from the dream state of mortality.

Sleeplessly, with adoring eyes, throughout the aeons of eternity I shall watch the lovely changes of expression on Thine infinite face.

I have dreamed many dreams I have dreamed many dreams; now I am awake. On my soul's altar I tend the sacred fire of constant remembrance of Thee. With my sleepless eyes of love I ever gaze on Thy face.

Through Thy grace I know that health and sickness, life and death, are but dreams. I have finished all stories of dreams, painted brightly and darkly on the world screen of delusion. Now I behold Thee as the only Reality.

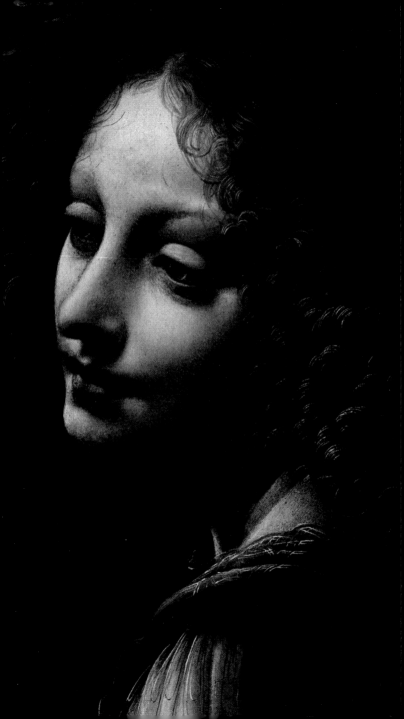

Thou didst teach me the language of angels

Incessantly searching, wandering through forests of Thy playful inaccessibility, at last I arrived at the portals of Infinity.

With faith and persistence I called Thy holy Name. The door of Thy dwelling opened. Within, on an altar of glorious visions, wert Thou, in perfect repose.

My ears were unattuned to Thy creation-molding voice; ardently but in vain I waited for Thee to speak. Gradually Thy spell of stillness stole over me, and in intuitional whispers Thou didst teach me the language of angels.

In the lisping tones of newborn communion I poured out my age-old questions: "Why, Lord, why sin and suffering? Why delusion?"

The rays of Thy shrine took form in letters of light and conveyed to me Thine answers—authentic, soul-solacing.

Now, in my chamber of inner peace, I am always at rest with Thee. We talk in words soundless, unknown to mortal hearing.

O Lord of the Unutterable Mysteries, ever in sacred silence shall We eloquently converse.

The rhythms of futurity

I disconnected the rays of my mind from the little territory of the senses and switched them on in the unrestricted land. The aurora of my attention spread in all directions.

Reality was no longer hidden behind flesh and appearances. I stood in unveiled regions and found streams of rushing, glistening thoughts. I felt the rippling currents of the millenniums—of born and unborn civilizations. In me all futurity danced in infinite rhythms.

I am Thy babe of eternity

Rocked in creation's cradle of past-present-future, I, Thy child of immortality, was restless.

Again and again I struggled ineffectually, but at last I managed to jump from the crib of delusive relativity. Thou didst catch me in Thine arms and rock me to eternal peace.

I am Thy babe of eternity, pillowed on Thy bosom of omnipresence.

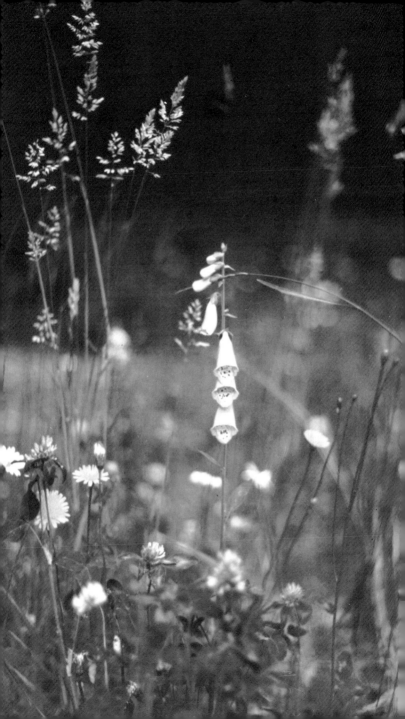

In my heart's patch of flowers   The bee of my mind makes its way to my heart's secluded garden, fanned by the breeze of my devotion and pearled with the dew of Thy sweetness.

I have grown for Thee stately lilies of discrimination, buttercup receptacles of my repentant tears, shy violets, dreaming of humility, and immense chrysanthemums of soul perceptions. To Thee my thought trees proffer on humble branch hands their fragrant fruit of prayer.

In my heart's patch of flowers my playful mind bee daily hovers, reveling among the nectared offerings to Thee.

O magic music of my soul!   In the wail of viols, in the humming of harps, and in the whisper sobs of my mind I caught echoes of Thee. Then I pulled down the stubborn veils of audible melodies. And, O Singer Infinite, I became aware of Thy voice! O Magic Music of my soul, at last I heard Thee!

Thou hast bestirred me from my age-old slumbers. Humbly I offer at Thine altar the bouquet of all my songs.

**Not against
my will,
O Death!**

I shall not be wrenched from the earth against my will, * like a truant boy pulled away from his playmates by his mother.

I love the Divine Mother; She loves me. When I go I shall have finished this role on the stage of time — that particular part which the Mother in Her cosmic vagaries longed to play through me.

Acting in the drama of life, I shall smile and weep—happy at fulfilled aspirations and anguished by shattered hopes. But when I have completed my assignment, however arduous, I shall depart with a laughing heart.

For a time I shall rest on the Mother's bosom of bliss; then return again to earth — not drawn here by past desires† unheedingly sown in the garden of delusion, but sent by Her soft command.

* The dramatic earth-exit of Paramahansa Yogananda took place in Los Angeles after he had uttered the concluding words in a speech of welcome to the Ambassador of India. The great master had long been aware that March 7, 1952, would be the date of his *mahasamadhi* (a yogi's conscious departure from the body). A memorial booklet, published by Self-Realization Fellowship, describes the closing days of his life. *(Publisher's Note)*

† See *reincarnation* in glossary.

"HELLO, PLAYMATE, I AM HERE!"

Alone I roamed the ocean shore,
And saw
   The wrestling waves in brawling roar,
Expressing Thine own restless life—
Thine angry mood in ripply quiver.
The violent vastness made me shiver
And turn away from Nature's strife.

And then
   A spreading sentinel tree
Waved friendly arms to comfort me,
With gentle look sublime.
Its swaying leaves in lull'by rhyme
A message sang I knew was Thine.

Above
   I scanned the gaugeless sky;
Within its bosom dim
I childlike tried on Thee to spy,
In play with Thee.

In vain I sought Thy body, hiding nigh,
Cloud-veiled, foam-sprayed, leaf-garlanded,
Too fine mine eyes to see;

Thy voice too pure mine ears to hear.
And yet
   I knew that Thou wert always near,
At hide-and-seek with me;
Receding, Spirit dear,
When almost I had touched the robe of Thee.

I groped for Thee through fold on fold
Of ignorance old, as time is old.
At last
   My search I stopped in dull despair,
My search for Thee, O Royal Sly Eluder!
    …everywhere,
Yet seeming nowhere…lost in unplumbed space,
Where none may clasp Thee nor behold Thy face.

In haste,
   I hied *away* from Thee.
Still, still no answer from the rageful sea,
And whispers only from the kindly tree;
Just silence from infinitudes of sky,
From valleys low and mountains high.
Hurt child, within the depths of me
I hid and sulked, not seeking Thee.

When lo!
   Unheralded, an Unseen Hand
Removed the maddening band

That blinded me in darkness old.
With joy untold
I turned and saw
A laughing sea, not one of wrathful roars;
A gay glad world, and open astral doors.

With only mists of dreams between,
Beside me *Someone* stood unseen,
And whispered to me, sweet and clear:
  "Hello, playmate! I am here!"

PARAMAHANSA YOGANANDA:
A YOGI IN LIFE AND DEATH

Paramahansa Yogananda entered *mahasamadhi* (a yogi's final conscious exit from the body) in Los Angeles, California, on March 7, 1952, after concluding his speech at a banquet held in honor of H. E. Binay R. Sen, Ambassador of India.

The great world teacher demonstrated the value of yoga (scientific techniques for God-realization) not only in life but in death. Weeks after his departure his unchanged face shone with the divine luster of incorruptibility.

Mr. Harry T. Rowe, Los Angeles Mortuary Director, Forest Lawn Memorial-Park (in which the body of the great master is temporarily placed), sent Self-Realization Fellowship a notarized letter from which the following extracts are taken:

"The absence of any visual signs of decay in the dead body of Paramahansa Yogananda offers the most extraordinary case in our experience.... No physical disintegration was visible in his body even twenty days after death.... No indication of mold was visible on his skin, and no visible desiccation (drying up) took place in the bodily tissues. This state of perfect preservation of a body is, so far as we know from mortuary annals, an unparalleled one.... At the time of receiving Yogananda's body, the Mortuary personnel expected to observe, through the glass lid of the casket, the usual progressive signs of bodily decay. Our astonishment increased as day followed day without bringing any visible change in the body under observation. Yogananda's body was apparently in a phenomenal state of immutability....

"No odor of decay emanated from his body at any time .... The physical appearance of Yogananda on March 27th, just before the bronze cover of the casket was put into position, was the same as it had been on March 7th. He looked on March 27th as fresh and as unravaged by decay as he had looked on the night of his death. On March 27th there was no reason to say that his body had suffered any visible physical disintegration at all. For these reasons we state again that the case of Paramahansa Yogananda is unique in our experience."

AIMS AND IDEALS
of
Self-Realization Fellowship

As set forth by Paramahansa Yogananda, Founder
Sri Daya Mata, President

To disseminate among the nations a knowledge of definite scientific techniques for attaining direct personal experience of God.

To teach that the purpose of life is the evolution, through self-effort, of man's limited mortal consciousness into God Consciousness; and to this end to establish Self-Realization Fellowship temples for God-communion throughout the world, and to encourage the establishment of individual temples of God in the homes and in the hearts of men.

To reveal the complete harmony and basic oneness of original Christianity as taught by Jesus Christ and original Yoga as taught by Bhagavan Krishna; and to show that these principles of truth are the common scientific foundation of all true religions.

To point out the one divine highway to which all paths of true religious beliefs eventually lead: the highway of daily, scientific, devotional meditation on God.

To liberate man from his threefold suffering: physical disease, mental inharmonies, and spiritual ignorance.

To encourage "plain living and high thinking"; and to spread a spirit of brotherhood among all peoples by teaching the eternal basis of their unity: kinship with God.

To demonstrate the superiority of mind over body, of soul over mind.

To overcome evil by good, sorrow by joy, cruelty by kindness, ignorance by wisdom.

To unite science and religion through realization of the unity of their underlying principles.

To advocate cultural and spiritual understanding between East and West, and the exchange of their finest distinctive features.

To serve mankind as one's larger Self.

GLOSSARY

Allah. Arabic word for God; the Name used by Moslems.

astral worlds. The subtle sphere of the Lord's creation, a universe of light composed of finer-than-atomic forces, i.e., vibrations of life energy or lifetrons (see *prana*). At physical death, the soul of man, clothed in its astral body of light, ascends to one of the planes of the astral "heaven," according to merit, to continue his spiritual evolution in the greater freedom of that subtle realm. There he remains for a karmically predetermined time until physical rebirth. (See *reincarnation.*)

Aum or **Om.** The basis of all sounds; universal symbol-word for God. *Aum* of the Vedas became the sacred word *Hum* of the Tibetans; *Amin* of the Moslems; and *Amen* of the Egyptians, Greeks, Romans, Jews, and Christians. *Amen* in Hebrew means *sure, faithful. Aum* is the all-pervading sound emanating from the Holy Ghost (Invisible Cosmic Vibration; God in His aspect of Creator); the "Word" of the Bible; the voice of creation, testifying to the Divine Presence in every atom. *Aum* may be heard through practice of Self-Realization Fellowship methods of meditation.

"These things saith the Amen, the faithful and true witness, the beginning of the creation of God." —Revelation 3:14. "In the beginning was the Word, and the Word was with God, and the Word was God....All things were made by him [the Word or *Aum*]; and without him was not any thing made that was made."—John 1:1, 3.

Babaji. See *Mahavatar Babaji.*

Bhagavad Gita. "Song of the Lord." This scripture, a part of the *Mahabharata* epic, consists of the sacred teachings of the avatar Lord Krishna as addressed to his chief disciple Arjuna.

Bhagavan Krishna. An avatar of India, a divine ruler of a mighty kingdom, approximately three millenniums before the Christian era. One of the meanings given for the word *Krishna* in the Hindu scriptures is "Omniscient Spirit." Thus, *Krishna*, like *Christ*, is a spiritual title signifying the divine magnitude of the avatar—his oneness with God. The title *Bhagavan* means "Lord." In his early life, Krishna lived as a cowherd who enchanted his companions with the music of his flute. In this role, Krishna represents allegorically the soul playing the flute of meditation to guide all misled thoughts back to the fold of omniscience.

Brahma. A Sanskrit word (from the root *brih*, to expand) for God in His aspect of Creator; Spirit as immanent in creation.

breath. "The influx of innumerable cosmic currents into man by way of the breath induces restlessness in his mind," Paramahansa Yogananda wrote. "Thus the breath links him with the fleeting phenomenal worlds. To escape from the sorrows of transitoriness and to enter the blissful realm of Reality, the yogi learns to quiet the breath by scientific meditation."

Buddha ("The Enlightened One"). One of the avatars of India; born in the 6th century B.C. at Kapilavastu.

Christ Consciousness. "Christ" or "Christ Consciousness" is the projected consciousness of God immanent in all creation. In Christian scripture it is called the "only begotten son," the only pure reflection in creation of God the Father. In Hindu scripture it is called *Kutastha Chaitanya* or *Tat,* the cosmic intelligence of Spirit everywhere present in creation. It is the universal consciousness, oneness with God, manifested by Jesus, Krishna, and other avatars. Great saints and yogis know it as the state of *samadhi* meditation wherein their consciousness has become identified with the intelligence in every particle of creation; they feel the entire universe as their own body. See *Sat-Tat-Aum.*

Cosmic Consciousness. The Absolute, beyond creation. Also the *samadhi*-meditation state of oneness with God both beyond and within vibratory creation. See *Sat-Tat-Aum.*

Cosmic Sound. See *Aum.*

Divine Mother. The aspect of God that is active in creation; the *shakti,* or power, of the Transcendent Creator. Other terms for this aspect of Divinity are *Aum, Shakti,* Holy Ghost, Cosmic Intelligent Vibration, Nature, Kali. Also, the personal aspect of God embodying the love and compassionate qualities of a mother.

The Hindu scriptures teach that God is both immanent and transcendent, personal and impersonal. He may be sought as the Absolute; as one of His manifest eternal qualities, such as love, wisdom, bliss, light; in the form of an *ishta* (deity); or as Father, Mother, or Friend.

egoism. The ego-principle, *ahamkara* (lit., "I do"), is the root cause of dualism or the seeming separation between man and his Creator. *Ahamkara* brings human beings under the sway of *maya (q.v.)*, by which the subject (ego) falsely appears as object; the creatures imagine themselves to be creators.

By banishing ego-consciousness, man awakens to his divine identity, his oneness with the Sole Life: God.

Gandhi, Mohandas K. ("Mahatma"). India's political saint, who in 1947 won freedom for India without war. He disciplined millions of Indians in the practices of nonviolent resistance to injustice. At various times in his life, because of his political activities, Gandhi was imprisoned. He was assassinated by a Hindu madman in New Delhi on January 30, 1948.

Gandhi wrote numerous books, including his famous autobiography, *The Story of My Experiments with Truth.* After his death, among thousands of other tributes, one from the Vatican in Rome read: "Gandhi is mourned as an apostle of Christian virtues." Albert Einstein said of the Mahatma: "Generations to come, it may be, will scarce believe that such a one as this ever in flesh and blood walked upon the earth."

gunas. The three attributes of Nature: *tamas, rajas,* and *sattva*—obstruction, activity, and expansion; or, mass, energy, and intelligence. In man the three *gunas* express themselves as ignorance or inertia; activity or struggle; and wisdom.

guru. When a devotee is ready to seek God in earnest, the Lord sends him a guru. Through the wisdom, intelligence, Self-realization, and teachings of such a master, God guides the disciple. By following the master's teachings and discipline, the disciple is able to fulfill his soul's desire for the manna of God-perception. A true guru, ordained by God to help sincere seekers in response to their deep soul craving, is not an ordinary teacher. He is a human vehicle whose body, speech, mind, and spirituality God uses as a channel to attract and guide lost souls back to their home of immortality. A guru is a living embodiment of scriptural truth. He is an agent of salvation appointed by God in response to a devotee's demand for release from the bondage of matter.

The term "guru" differs from "teacher," as a person may have many teachers but only one guru.

Hindu. A member of one of the ancient races of India who follows the teachings of Hinduism (which embraces various religious systems based on four profound scriptures, the Vedas—*q.v.*).

holy vibration. See *Aum*.

intuition. The "sixth sense"; apprehension of knowledge derived immediately and spontaneously from the soul, not from the fallible medium of the senses or of reason.

ji. A suffix denoting respect, added to names and titles in India; as, Gandhiji, Paramahansaji, guruji.

Kali. God in His aspect of Nature—the Cosmic Mother. In Hindu art She is represented as four-armed. One of the divine hands symbolizes Her powers of creation; the second hand, the universal principle of preservation; the third hand, the purifying forces of dissolution. Kali's fourth hand is outstretched in a gesture of blessing and salvation. In this fourfold way She leads all creation back to its source in Spirit.

karma. "Action," or specifically, the effects of past actions, from this or previous lifetimes. The equilibrating law of karma, as expounded in the Hindu scriptures, is that of action and reaction, cause and effect, sowing and reaping. In the course of natural righteousness, each man by his thoughts and actions becomes the molder of his destiny. Whatever energies he himself, wisely or unwisely, has set in motion must return to him as their starting point, like a circle inexorably completing itself. "The world looks like a mathematical equation, which, turn it how you will, balances itself. Every secret is told, every crime is punished, every virtue rewarded, every wrong redressed, in silence and certainty" (Emerson, in *Compensation*). An understanding of karma as the law of justice serves to free the human mind from resentment against God and man. See *reincarnation.*

Koran. The holy scripture of Islam.

Krishna. See *Bhagavan Krishna.*

Kriya Yoga. A sacred spiritual science, originating millenniums ago in India. It includes certain techniques of meditation whose devoted practice leads to realization of God. Kriya Yoga is praised by Krishna in the Bhagavad Gita and by Patanjali in the *Yoga Sutras*. Revived in this age by Mahavatar Babaji (*q.v.*), Kriya Yoga is the spiritual initiation bestowed by the Gurus of Self-Realization Fellowship on qualified students of the *Self-Realization Lessons* (see page 213).

Lahiri Mahasaya. *Lahiri* was the family name of Shyama Charan Lahiri (1828–1895). *Mahasaya,* a Sanskrit religious title, means "large-minded." Lahiri Mahasaya was a disciple of Mahavatar Babaji, and the guru of Swami Sri Yukteswar (Paramahansa Yogananda's guru). A Christlike teacher with miraculous powers, he was also a family man with business responsibilities. His mission was to make known a yoga suitable for modern man, in which meditation is balanced by right performance of worldly duties. Lahiri Mahasaya is referred to as a *Yogavatar,* "Incarnation of Yoga." He was the disciple to whom Babaji revealed the ancient, almost lost science of Kriya Yoga *(q.v.),* instructing him in turn to initiate sincere seekers. Lahiri Mahasaya's life is described in *Autobiography of a Yogi.*

Mahavatar Babaji. The deathless *mahavatar* ("great avatar") who in 1861 gave Kriya Yoga initiation to Lahiri Mahasaya, and thereby restored to the world this ancient technique of salvation. More information about his life and spiritual mission is given in *Autobiography of a Yogi.*

maya. The delusory power inherent in the structure of creation, by which the One appears as many. *Maya* is the principle of relativity, inversion, contrast, duality, oppositional states; the "Satan" (lit., in Hebrew, "the adversary") of the Old Testament prophets; and the "devil" whom Christ described picturesquely as a "murderer" and a "liar,'" because "there is no truth in him" (John 8:44). Paramahansa Yogananda wrote:

"The Sanskrit word *maya* means 'the measurer'; it is the magical power in creation by which limitations and divisions are apparently present in the Immeasurable and Inseparable. *Maya* is Nature herself—the phenomenal worlds, ever in transitional flux as antithesis to Divine Immutability.

"In God's plan and play *(lila)*, the sole function of Satan or *Maya* is to attempt to divert man from Spirit to matter, from Reality to unreality. 'The devil sinneth from the beginning. For this purpose the Son of God was manifested, that he might destroy the works of the devil.' (I John 3:8). That is, the manifestation of Christ Consciousness, within man's own being, effortlessly destroys the illusions or 'works of the devil.'

"*Maya* is the veil of transitoriness in Nature, the ceaseless becoming of creation; the veil that each man must lift in order to see behind it the Creator, the changeless immutable eternal Reality."

meditation. Generally, interiorized concentration with the objective of perceiving God. True meditation, *dhyana*, is conscious realization of God through intuitive perception. It is achieved only after the devotee has attained that fixed concentration whereby he has disconnected his attention from the senses and is completely undisturbed by sensory perceptions from the outer world. Perfected meditation deepens into the state of *samadhi, (q.v.),* communion, oneness with God.

Mohammed. Seventh-century prophet; the great founder of Islam.

Nanak. Medieval leader and illumined saint of the Sikhs in India.

pagoda. A towerlike temple or memorial, common in India, China, and Japan. The pyramidal stone pagodas of India are among the finest examples of temple architecture. Chinese pagodas, usually made of brick, have a small rooflike projection at each successive story.

paramahansa. A spiritual title signifying one who is master of himself. It may be conferred only by a true guru on a qualified disciple. In the Hindu scriptures, the *hansa* or swan symbolizes spiritual discrimination. *Parama* means "supreme."

prana. Cosmic life force in the human body and in all living creatures.

Rama. An ancient avatar of India; central figure in the sacred epic, *Ramayana.*

Ramprasad (1718-1775). A Bengali saint who composed many songs in praise of Kali *(q.v.),* one of the aspects of the Divine Mother.

reincarnation. The doctrine set forth in the Hindu scriptures that human beings, entangled in a web of unfulfilled desires, are forced to return again and again to earth. When man consciously regains his true status as a son of God, the otherwise inexorable cycle of reincarnation ceases. "Him that overcometh will I make a pillar in the temple of my God, and he shall go no more out."—Rev. 3:12. Understanding of the law of karma and of its corollary, reincarnation, is implicit in many Bible passages.

The early Christian Church accepted the doctrine of reincarnation, which was expounded by the Gnostics and by numerous Church fathers, including Clement of Alexandria, the celebrated Origen, and the fifth-century St. Jerome. The theory was first declared a heresy in A.D. 553 by the Second Council of Constantinople. At that time many Christians thought the doctrine of reincarnation afforded man too ample a stage of time and space to encourage him to strive for immediate salvation. Today many Western thinkers accept the theories of karma and reincarnation, seeing in them the laws of justice that underlie life's seeming inequalities. See *karma.*

samadhi. Superconsciousness. *Samadhi* is attained by following the eightfold path outlined in the *Yoga Sutras* by the great ancient authority, Patanjali. *Samadhi* is the eighth step or final goal. Scientific meditation (the right use of yoga techniques developed millenniums ago by India's *rishis,* sages) leads the devotee to *samadhi* or God-realization. As the wave melts in the sea, so the human soul realizes itself as omnipresent Spirit.

Sat-Tat-Aum. Father, Son, and Holy Ghost; or, God in the aspect of the Father: transcendent or *nirguna,* "without qualities"—Cosmic Consciousness in the blissful void *beyond* creation, beyond the phenomenal worlds; God in the aspect of the Son: Christ Consciousness, immanent in creation; and God in the aspect of the Holy Ghost: *Aum (q.v.),* the Divine Creative Vibration.

Self-Realization Fellowship (SRF). The society founded by Paramahansa Yogananda in 1920 (and as Yogoda Satsanga Society of India in 1917) to disseminate worldwide, through the *Self-Realization Lessons,* the spiritual principles and techniques of Kriya Yoga for the aid and benefit of humanity. Sri Daya Mata, one of the foremost direct disciples of Paramahansa Yogananda, is the current SRF/YSS president.

The international headquarters, the Mother Center, is in Los Angeles, California. Here, monks and nuns of the Self-Realization Order carry on many activities to serve the worldwide membership of SRF, including publication of the *SRF Lessons,* books, recordings, and *Self-Realization Magazine,* which contains previously unpublished lectures and writings of Paramahansa Yogananda. SRF directs a Voluntary League whose members supply food and clothing to the needy in various parts of the world. The SRF Worldwide Prayer Circle, composed of men and women in many lands, daily prays for world peace and sends healing vibrations to all who request help in freeing themselves from physical disease, mental inharmonies, and spiritual ignorance.

Paramahansa Yogananda has explained the meaning of the organization's name in this way: "Self-Realization Fellowship signifies fellowship with God through Self-realization, and friendship with all truth-seeking souls." See also "Aims and Ideals of Self-Realization Fellowship," page 202.

Self-Realization Order. The monastic branch of Self-Realization Fellowship, created by Paramahansa Yogananda and charged with the responsibility of carrying out his wishes for the guidance and spiritual welfare of Self-Realization Fellowship and its worldwide membership.

Shankara, Swami. Sometimes referred to as Adi ("the first") Shankaracharya (Shankara + *acharya,* "teacher"). India's most illustrious philosopher. His date is uncertain; many scholars assign him to the ninth century. He expounded God not as a negative abstraction but as positive, eternal, omnipresent, ever-new Bliss. Shankara reorganized the ancient Swami Order, and founded four great *maths* (monastic centers of spiritual education), whose leaders in apostolic succession bear the title Jagadguru Sri Shankaracharya. The meaning of *Jagadguru* is "world teacher."

Shiva. The aspect of the Infinite Transcendental Spirit that exists in relation to Its "consort" Kali *(q.v.)* — the finite world of Nature.

spiritual eye. The "single" eye of wisdom, the pranic star door through which man must enter to attain Cosmic Consciousness. The method of entering the sacred door is taught by Self-Realization Fellowship.

In the Hindu scriptures the forehead in man is called the "eastern" part of his body — a divine microcosm. The single eye of omniscience is located in the forehead between the two eyebrows.

"I am the door: by me if any man enter in, he shall be saved, and shall go in and out, and find pasture."—John 10:9. "When thine eye is single, thy whole body also is full of light....Take heed, therefore, that the light which is in thee be not darkness."—Luke 11:34–35.

Sri Yukteswar, Swami (1855–1936). The great guru of Paramahansa Yogananda, who called him *Jnanavatar* or "Incarnation of Wisdom." Sri Yukteswar's beautiful life is described in Paramahansaji's *Autobiography of a Yogi.*

Swami. A member of India's most ancient monastic order, reorganized in the eighth century by Swami

Shankara *(q.v.)*. A swami takes formal vows of celibacy and renunciation of worldly ambitions; he devotes himself to meditation and service to humanity. There are ten classificatory titles of the venerable Swami Order, as *Giri, Puri, Bharati, Tirtha, Saraswati,* and others. Swami Sri Yukteswar *(q.v.)* and Paramahansa Yogananda belonged to the *Giri* ("mountain") branch.

The Sanskrit word *swami* means "he who is one with the Self *(Swa)*."

Vedas. The four scriptural texts of the Hindus: *Rig Veda, Sama Veda, Yajur Veda,* and *Atharva Veda.* They are essentially a literature of chant and recitation. Among the immense texts of India, the Vedas (Sanskrit root *vid,* to know) are the only writings to which no author is ascribed. The *Rig Veda* assigns a celestial origin to the hymns and tells us they have come down from "ancient times," reclothed in new language. Divinely revealed from age to age to the *rishis,* "seers," the four Vedas are said to possess *nityatva,* "timeless finality."

vihara. The temple and grounds of monasteries of the Buddhists and Jains.

yoga. From Sanskrit *yuj,* "union." The highest connotation of the word *yoga* in Hindu philosophy is union of the individual soul with Spirit through scientific methods of meditation. There are various yoga methods: *Hatha Yoga, Mantra Yoga, Laya Yoga, Karma Yoga, Jnana Yoga, Bhakti Yoga,* and *Raja Yoga. Raja Yoga,* the "royal" or complete yoga, is the scientific path taught by Self-Realization Fellowship; it includes the highest aspects of all other forms of yoga.

yogi. One who practices yoga. Anyone who practices a scientific technique for divine realization is a yogi. Yogis may be either married or unmarried; they may take on worldly responsibilities or formal religious vows.

Yogoda Satsanga Society of India. The name by which Self-Realization Fellowship is known in India. The society was founded in 1917 by Paramahansa Yogananda. Its headquarters, Yogoda Math, is situated on the banks of the Ganges at Dakshineswar, near Calcutta. Yogoda Satsanga Society has a branch *math* at Ranchi, Bihar, and many branch centers throughout India. In addition to Yogoda meditation centers and groups, the society has twenty-two educational institutions, from primary through college standard. The literal meaning of *Yogoda,* a word coined by Paramahansa Yogananda, is "that which yoga imparts," i.e., Self-realization. *Satsanga* means "divine fellowship," or "fellowship with God, or truth." For the West, Paramahansaji translated the Indian name as "Self-Realization Fellowship"*(q.v.)*.

yuga. A cycle or subperiod of creation, outlined in ancient Hindu texts. In *The Holy Science,* a book in English by Sri Yukteswar *(q.v.)*, he describes a 24,000-year Equinoctial Cycle and mankind's present place in it.

A "Day of Creation" is said to be four billion years; "One Age of Brahma" or the life span of a whole universe is given as 314 trillion years.

ALPHABETICAL INDEX OF TITLES

Adoring Thee through all the aeons 190
Affirmation for healing others 86
All creation is Thine inimitable handiwork......... 90
All power is divine...100
An ever present Sentry of Light 13
At play with Thee..163
At Thy touch, dumb matter speaks 177
Aum, the heartbeat of creation 52
Awake and ready...182
Beauty of Thy plan, The..182
"Be happy, My child!" 152
Be my Captain 102
Be Thou my Beacon of Wisdom 69
Be Thou my Sun and Moon 42
Be Thou President of a United World......................64
Bless me, that my five senses encounter
    only goodness...116
Blow through the flute of my being........................ 89
Blue-rayed lotus of Thy feet, The.........................155
Boom Thou on the shores of my mind 75
Butterfly of eternity, A 183
By trials may I perfect myself 70
Caravan of my prayers is moving onward, The 117
Come, O Perfect Joy!..103
Come out of the cocoon of delusion........................107
Come to me as Buddha...136
Come to me as Mohammed 134
Come to me as Moses 133
Come to me as Swami Shankara 132
Come to me in a tangible human form 107
Come to me, O Christ, as the Good Shepherd 129
Come to me, O Krishna, as the Divine Cowherd....131

Correct my defective vision 101
Crying in the wilderness... 24
Darkness vanishes before Thy light........................121
Death's reply 36
Destroying the fortress of ignorance 39
Devotee's aspiration, The 40
Devotee's vow, The..123
Dewdrops of repentance.. 87
Diving for the Pearl of Great Price 83
Divine Sculptor, The 29
Doors everywhere 158
Dreaming, I thought I was awake 165
Each of us reflects Thine individuality 61
Ego, the impersonator 103
Fivefold taper of my senses, The 38
Forest of delusion ablaze, The................................185
Forget me not, though I forget Thee........................ 96
For Thee: a bouquet of all loves 76
From joy I came, for joy I live.................................. 97
Gandhi, the Mahatma—"great soul" 137
Gaze of truth, The.. 81
Give me fervor in divine love 16
Give me the humblest place within Thy heart 9
Give us a true conception of brotherhood 54
Giving smiles to everyone.......................................143
Glance Thou into my ardent eyes 61
God alone! 31
Guard me from highway robbers............................. 49
Guide me, O Soul Charioteer!.................................108
Happiness is our birthright......................................110
Hasten Thou the day 122
Heal us in body, mind, and soul.............................. 86
Healing affirmation.. 86
Heavenly Hart, I hunted Thee in the forest
   of consciousness... 90
Heavenly Thief of Hearts 73
"Hello, playmate, I am here!" (poem) 197

Help me to win the battle of life................................109
Honeycomb of my heart, The 174
I adore Thee in the language of love.........................116
I am a spark of Thy cosmic fire.............................. 62
I am a wave of joy.. 74
I am building a rainbow bridge to reach Thee..........104
I am Homeward bound at last 39
I am immortal Spirit.. 94
I am Thy babe of eternity 193
I am Thy bird of paradise 106
I am Thy divine dewdrop..100
I am Thy tiny hummingbird   9
I asked Thee: "What is sin?".....................................167
I beheld Thee hiding in a flower 158
I beheld Thee in Thy dances of creation,
    preservation, and destruction 178
I bow to Thee everywhere 146
I come with the myrrh of reverence........................ 53
I fly from life to life... 78
I have dreamed many dreams 190
I heard Thy gentle voice saying: "Come Home"...... 49
Immortalizing rays of Spirit, The.............................168
In appearance, many; in essence, One..................... 19
Infinitude's happy child... 44
In my heart's patch of flowers.................................195
Inspirit us with generosity 20
In the bursts of blue brine 162
In the garden of my life... 118
In the nightly garden of dreams 35
Invincible Lion of the Self..175
I play hide-and-seek with Thee................................164
I remember, I remember! 162
I shall be a messenger of joy 164
I shall spread Thy holy Name 174
I shall swim in the sea of souls................................173
I swept Thy wisdom's ocean for treasure 189
I valiantly struggle toward Thee............................... 95

I was shipwrecked on the ocean of life 51
I wear my scars as roses of courage..........................161
I will be Thine always 85
I will be Thy naughty baby, O Divine Mother! 111
I yearn to hear Thy unique voice............................. 11
Keep me away from evil..112
Lark that drinks Thy raindrops, The.........................184
Lead me to the royal highway of realization 112
Let all rest in the shade of my peace 169
Lord's Prayer: a humble interpretation, The............ 56
Make me a smile millionaire 63
Make me clean again, Divine Mother...................... 24
Master Mariner, take charge of my boat.................. 94
May cocktails of devotion induce God-intoxication 42
May human love become divine love 13
May I abandon the anger habit................................. 77
May I act from free choice, not habit 10
May I be cheerfully busy 51
May I calm the storms of restless desires 68
May I discipline the senses 82
May I drown in Thine Ocean and live...................... 57
May I exude only sweetness 112
May I find my Self in all... 71
May I find Thy love in all 145
May I forgive all 6
May I help, not punish, wrongdoers......................... 62
May I live less by food and more by cosmic light....101
May I love Thee as saints love Thee 11
May I make others happy 143
May I overcome fear... 50
May I reap the harvest of Cosmic Consciousness .. 43
May I savor with Thy zest all innocent pleasures... 78
May I see goodness in others 42
May I still the gale of passions 60
May my gratitude be changeless 85
May my love for Thee be unfading............................110
May our hearts repeat Thy name 113

Meditation and devotion.. 73
Melody of human brotherhood, The 3
Memories 155
Misleading folly fires 102
My Guru, Sri Yukteswar 128
My Home is Heaven..146
My journey's end 177
My taper of remembrance of Thee......................... 95
Nightingale of heaven, A 173
Not against my will, O Death! 196
O Colossal Denizen of the Deeps! 166
O Fairy Song of Love Everlasting! 152
O Lord, our first duty is to Thee 33
O magic music of my soul! 195
Open the petaled bars of our heart buds 35
O Spirit, I worship Thee in all shrines 19
O Spirit, reveal Thyself as Thou art......................114
Our purified rivers reach Thy Sea......................... 59
Overcoming my enemies: bad habits 109
O Virtue! thou art infinitely more charming
     than Vice.. 87
O Wine of Centuries!..156
Prayer at dawn.. 66
Prayer at eventide... 67
Prayer at night.. 67
Prayer at noon 66
Prayer before meditation 16
Prayer before taking food 123
Prayer for peace.. 93
Prayer for supply of immediate needs....................119
Prayer for the Great Enlightenment 122
Prayer of loyalty, A 160
Prayer of my heart.. 81
Prayer to the Holy Trinity 99
Prince of peace, sitting on the throne of poise, A ... 40
Purify me in a furnace of trials 97
Remove Thou the veils of creation 59

Removing the cork of ignorance 163
Removing the debris of delusion 106
Repair my nerve wires, O Mystic Electrician!........ 96
Restore our transparency 113
Revive my friendship with Thee 102
Rhythms of futurity, The..193
Right thinking for prosperity 69
River of ardor, A.. 24
Salutation to God as the Great Preceptor   3
Salutation to Spirit..111
Save me from sense slavery 17
Save me from wrong beliefs 95
Save us from the dragnet of delusion 83
Seraphic strains of *Aum*, The 157
Spiritualize us, O Infinite Alchemist! 99
Star that leads to the Christ Child, The................... 15
Stricken are here at Thy door, The 47
Sun gaze of my love ne'er sets, The........................ 89
Taper of meditation, The.. 46
Tell me Thou hast loved me always 33
Tell me—wilt Thou be mine?.................................. 21
Terrors of mundane delusion are but dreams 172
Thine approaching feet 189
Thine eagle of soul progress..................................... 45
Thine is the Sole Life 29
Thou art ever busy, O Cosmic Potter! 22
Thou art hiding behind a veil of cosmic rays......... 82
Thou art Love..144
Thou art my Best Friend 145
Thou art my Protector 53
Thou art my Well-Wisher 141
Thou art Peace and Silence......................................141
Thou art plainly present 143
Thou art the Cause of all..144
Thou art the Fountain of Love..................................153
Thou art the highest goal of man............................. 45
Thou art the Sole Doer 63

Thou art visible as Mother Nature 26
Thou didst baptize me in the flood of Thy grace.....157
Thou didst teach me the language of angels 192
Thou dost ever behold me 119
Thought at Christmas... 54
Thou hast many Names 118
Thou hast no body..144
Thou hast satisfied my soul hunger 183
Thou lookest for my coming................................... 52
Thy *danse macabre* 169
Thy light in the sunless ocean depths 160
Thy light transfigures all creation.......................... 15
Thy magnum opus of *Aum* 73
Thy pristine song gushed through me 186
Thy simple song of joy..117
Thy station, JOY...186
Unbroken oneness 80
Universal daily prayer for divine guidance 109
Untutored song of my heart, The 21
Vision of Christ and Krishna, A 170
We are actors in Thy cosmic pictures 92
We are Thy burned children, wailing for Thy help.. 80
We demand as Thy children.................................... 47
Welcome, O Majestic Personage!............................153
We unite to worship Thee, O Spirit! 4
What bliss at the sight of Thy light! 185
Whispers from Eternity 151
Why dost Thou seem so far away? 120
Wondrous eyes of Christ, The 188